love the cover of ... walnut?

Be well —

[signature] Skookumtumtum

Uncle Steve

April

2012

THE RANCID WALNUT: AN ULTRARUNNING PSYCHOLOGIST'S JOURNEY WITH PROSTATE CANCER

R. Steven Heaps, Ph.D. ("Skookumtumtum")

"The Rancid Walnut: An Ultrarunning Psychologist's Journey With Prostate Cancer" by R. Steven Heaps, Ph. D. ISBN 978-1-60264-994-1 (softcover) ISBN 978-1-62137-008-6 (electronic copy).

Library of Congress Control Number: 2012904963

Published 2012 by Virtualbookworm.com Publishing Inc., P.O. Box 9949, College Station, TX 77842, US. © 2012, R. Steven Heaps, Ph. D.

Manufactured in the United States of America.

On a sunny, spring day in 1961, I was driving down the hill on Rowan Avenue. When I honked and waved at a gorgeous 15-year old blonde, she smiled and returned my wave. We went to a movie two nights later, and she has been with me ever since.

When a spouse has a serious illness, there is no substitute for a devoted, loving partner. I am grateful to have lived my life with Karen. This book is dedicated to her.

ACKNOWLEDGEMENTS

My urologist and surgeon, Robert Golden, M.D., and my psychologist friend, Dennis Dyck, Ph.D., Vice Chancellor of Research at Washington State University, read an early draft of this book to verify the accuracy of its medical and psychological information, respectively. Their enthusiasm helped me to persevere with this project. Thanks also to Rob for writing the Foreword.

My second cousin, Gary Maxwell, M.D., and community college English instructor, Mark Doerr, offered useful comments on the beginning chapters. Gary's son, Brian, and his wife, Jen Liu, both resident physicians at Stanford University, took time from their hectic schedules to contribute their medical opinions.

My graduate school mentor and long-time friend, Richard Powers, Ph.D., completed a critique that was even more extensive than the one he furnished for my dissertation in 1974. His suggestions enabled me to create a more coherent story.

Marilyn Schuster Rowan, long-time English teacher, functioned as my FGoVU ("Fairy Godmother of Verbal Usage"), and in the process went from being a high school acquaintance, to being a friend. Her input saved me from untold grammatical transgressions.

Steve Merryman from SIGMA created the design for the book cover. The artwork is not only of high quality, but it makes me laugh.

For fear of omitting someone's name, I will avoid listing the numerous friends who gave me support and encouragement. I'll get around to thanking them all in person, and they know who they are.

My dear sister, Lynne, has championed everything I have ever attempted. Her writing talent combined with her passionate interest in my work has inspired me.

My children and grandchildren help give meaning to my life. Time with them is a treasure for me. I appreciate the fact that I have the good fortune to be surrounded by people like them who love me. Steven, Sue, Heather, Dwain, Kaitlyn and McKenzie—I love you guys.

And then there is my wife, Karen, who read and proof-read every word of this book, and functioned as a patient sounding board. Her love throughout this project was, as usual, the rock-solid center of my life.

TABLE OF CONTENTS

FOREWORD

When the diagnosis of prostate cancer enters the life of an experienced psychologist, a world of unease, desperation and rapid exploration ensues. The journey transcends the denial, anger, bargaining and acceptance of an unwelcome event in your life. Prostate cancer exposes our mortality, priorities, vulnerability and ultimate sense of being. The all-consuming questions of who am I, what do I want and why am I here are thrust front and center.

Steve Heaps' journey of discovery, research, decision, therapy and acceptance is one of courage and openness. His willingness to learn, inquire and follow through exemplify an honest man of principle.

For some reason, I was gifted the honor of guiding Dr. Heaps through the brambles and confusion of the options for treatment and non-treatment of his prostate cancer. Our discussions were enlightening for me. Steve and his wife, Karen, were present at every turn, asking probing questions and following up with even more insight into the disease. It is these decisions that highlight the growth and discovery of self. Steve invites us to share in this discovery.

There are layers of insight in *The Rancid Walnut*. The gathering of information about options for therapy is a challenge in itself. The exact choice of therapy is not as important as the process of becoming comfortable with the decision. There is no right or wrong way to treat localized prostate cancer. What is important is that the decision you make is one you can live with, knowing you looked at all the risks and benefits of the therapy. Steve's choice of therapy and following through with its completion really was just the beginning of his journey of acceptance. Even to this day, there are decisions, worries and ongoing acceptance of what is. And, it is this living day-to-day with the questions which allows us to be present and grow our gratitude for ourselves, family, friends and connection.

The Rancid Walnut is both educational and touching. We are always learning new angles of viewing the seemingly complex world of prostate cancer. This book is a whole new take on the unique adventure of being diagnosed with prostate cancer. Enjoy and read with an open heart.

Rob Golden, M.D.

PREFACE

This book belongs to the genre known as memoir, creative non-fiction, or personal essay. I have made a serious attempt to be accurate and truthful. Given the vagaries of memory, that goal can never be perfectly met. When I am using some degree of poetic license to fill in the details, I'll let you know. In his informative book, *Writing Life Stories*, Bill Roorbach notes that when Terry Gross was interviewing author David Sedaris on the National Public Radio program *Fresh Air*, she asked him how true his memoirs are. He said, simply, "True enough."

I hope what follows is "true enough."

Some who are a part of my story are identified. Others, for reasons of the privacy of their reactions or experiences, are without attribution. If you recognize yourself or someone else herein, you may or may not be correct.

1

DIAGNOSIS

Each man will engage prostate cancer in his own fashion. Regardless of our health status, every day brings things that need to be done. For decades, I have organized my daily life by creating To Do lists. These columns of tasks scribbled on 3X5 note cards or the kitchen whiteboard, though never completely finished, provide order to my world. They create a sense of control over life, even when the most important things are beyond control.

To Do lists are most effective when used to rank activities by order of importance, since it is so tempting to tackle the easier items first. However, stressful events often disrupt this strategy. Adversity prompts actions that distract people from negative experiences such as worry, fear, and a sense of loss of control. The resulting behaviors can take on comical, even absurd qualities.

Join me in real life during the winter of 2008. Consider the To Do list on the next page:

TO DO LIST

1. Have cancerous prostate removed.
2. Call about insurance.
3. Buy dog food.
4. Check tire pressure on truck.
5. Write thank you notes.
6. Hang up clothes.
7. Rearrange furniture.

It's 3 a.m. as I hoist the hide-a-bed up on end, and it jams in the doorway, trapping me in the office next to the family room. I wrestle it back far enough to squeeze by and make it to the garage. Shivering in my underwear, I pad bare footed across the January-cold concrete to fetch a hammer and nail to remove the door. There's room now to shove the bed through. Or there was, until the bed springs open and slams the side of my head, pinning my neck to the door frame.

While I mutter to myself, Karen observes silently in non-sidewalk-superintendent mode. I think she knows that this is a good time to let my obsessive-compulsiveness run its course. Of course, now the basement door also needs to come off to provide additional space. It mashes my big toe. Pushing and grunting, pulling and cursing, I eventually maneuver the bed into the space I had created amidst the family room furniture.

Karen must have some reservations about this domestic realignment. At a bare minimum, she has to be questioning my timing. True, she moves the furniture several times per year, usually when I'm out of town and always during daylight hours. I have never been able to fathom why she would go to all that effort. We'd had a number of discussions about the hide-a-bed. I'd changed my mind or had it changed by her several times. Finally, last week we'd agreed to leave it where it was. I'd recuperate on the sofa. This morning, though, the hide-a-bed absolutely must travel to the family room.

We are getting ready to leave for the hospital, where I will undergo a prostatectomy. I had been telling Karen and myself that I was worried about climbing to the master bedroom on the second floor during my recovery, and that I thought that lying on the hide-a-bed would also prevent Hershey, our Chocolate Lab, from flopping his 95 pounds on top of me—yeah, it's Hershey's fault, and he didn't even bother to come down to see what I was doing, let alone to lend a paw.

Maybe I also want the hide-a-bed out there for symbolic support, since we had purchased it for Dad to sleep on, so that he did not have to deal with our stairs up to the bedrooms. Or maybe it's because it was on the edge of this bed that I sat up with him most of the night before the day his aneurism burst. However, in my heart of hearts, I know now that my frantic struggle here is, instead, a last gasp at trying to be in control of something, anything, in the face of a situation in which I will have very little control.

"Is this Mr. Heaps?" "Yes."

"This is Dr. Rinaldi's office calling. He'd like you to make an appointment to see him."

I respond, "Oh, so my PSA must have gone up. You wouldn't be calling me to come in if he wanted to tell me about my cholesterol levels."

The PSA test is a tool frequently used as an initial screen for the presence of prostate cancer. This test measures the amount of prostate specific antigen, an enzyme produced in the prostate and normally found in the blood. Its level is affected by a variety of conditions, only one of which is cancer; thus, high PSA scores do not necessarily indicate the presence of that disease. Prostatitis (inflammation of the prostate), benign prostatic hypertrophy (enlargement of the prostate that causes problems with urination), ejaculation within the 48 hours preceding the test, and localized trauma, such as from a bicycle seat, are common causes of an elevated PSA. Also, some people just naturally produce more of this particular antigen. For example, I have a friend who is in his late 70s, and who for decades has recorded PSA scores into the high teens, yet there has been no indication that he has prostate cancer.

I'd had the lab do a PSA test when I recently had my blood drawn for a cholesterol check. Two tests with only one blood draw saved me one stick in the arm. I enjoy being poked even less than previously, after a phlebotomist at a different lab stabbed a needle clear through a vein and destroyed it. I had been first in line that morning. Maybe she was hung over. Maybe she'd had a fight with a skinny boyfriend with a big nose. Or maybe it was just the luck of the draw, but I ended up with two solid, ropy bulges in place of a smooth vein, and no blood flows past this blockage. Dr. Rinaldi said not to worry about it, that to try to fix it would probably make things worse, and anyway, I had a lot of collateral vessels to do the job. I was tempted to say, "Yeah, that's easy for you to say. It's not your arm." But I kept my mouth shut for once. I just made sure to have my blood drawn at his office, rather than at the lab.

After making the appointment, I remembered that a year ago I had also gotten a single blood draw for the cholesterol and the PSA, and the cardiologist's office had called with my cholesterol numbers, and told me incidentally that my PSA had increased from 3.6 to 4.5. For years, a PSA value above 4.0 had been considered abnormal. There has been an ongoing debate as to the cut-off level, and it now seems that the rate at which the level is rising is more important than its absolute value. The cardiologist's office asked if my primary care doctor had asked to see me. I said he hadn't. At that point, I took no follow-up action. A mistake? An example of my hating to be told what to do? Could be. I sometimes have an immediate, irrational reaction when I think someone is telling me what to do. I don't know. I'm working, albeit with limited success, on not second-guessing myself.

We have been exceedingly fortunate to have Peter Rinaldi as our family doctor for over 30 years. We met him when Dick Groesbeck and I began our psychology practice in the same complex where Pete had started his family practice a few months earlier, gradually building a reputation as one of the finest primary care doctors in the area. He had referred patients to me for psychotherapy consistently for the 28 years I was in practice. He's an avid big game hunter and a truly nice guy. I respect him. I like him. I trust him.

When I went in, he said that my PSA had increased to 6.9, but noted that a rising PSA did not necessarily signify trouble. "I doubt if there is a problem, but we need to check. I never go by just the PSA. I rely on both the PSA level and the physical exam, the digital rectal exam. After a while, you get so that you can tell things just by feel from the exam," he explained.

I know that many of you guys find it embarrassing to go in for a rectal exam. You might even skip checkups because you don't want some guy, doctor or not, sticking his finger up your rear. If you have a female doctor, you probably aren't too hot about her overly personal explorations either.

Events are most humorous when they contain an element of truth. We often handle things that scare or embarrass us through humor. Recently on the radio, I heard Ray Romano from *Everybody Loves Raymond* reporting that Hallmark even had a card for the occasion of turning forty that read, "Happy Birthday! Bend Over." Describing his unease, he said, "I was afraid it would hurt." Following a comedic pause, he added, "And then I was more afraid that it wouldn't." The last comment evoked the most laughter.

What if the comedian's second feared outcome occurred? What if the rectal exam actually felt somewhat pleasurable? Such an outcome says nothing about a man being gay. The body is just responding to a particular form of stimulation. After all, contractions of the prostate are part of what makes a man's orgasm pleasurable. The rectal exam is just that, an exam. I say, "Get over it."

I recall my first awareness of my body responding sexually. Go back with me to Spokane, Washington, in 1955. I'm eleven years old and late for dinner on a December evening. As I speed my sled down the icy hill on Bismarck Place for yet another "final run" in the fading daylight, the snow is slapping me in the face and my eyes sting. I close my eyes but am so fearful of being smashed by one of the cars driving across the arterial at the bottom that I keep popping them open, and they fill with snow, so I'm flying blind anyway. *What's this?* My sled is rattling over the frozen ruts in the road, and the vibration on my pubic bone feels good. No, it doesn't feel good; it feels great. *What's that all about?* When I skid to a stop at Driscoll Boulevard, I leap from my sled and look around to see if anyone is looking at me funny. Two younger girls I don't know are trailing after their yammering mother toward the open tailgate of a green station wagon. My friend, Mike, is already half way back up the hill. I race after him, slipping and sliding, falling twice before I reach the top. I'm going to catch it from Mom for being late, and I have no idea what the hell is happening to me, but I'm certainly going to try to make it happen at least one more time before I head home for dinner.

So that's how I remember it after 57 years. Whether some of the details are be-fogged by time isn't as important as what my experience says about our sexual responses. I don't recall linking my bodily sensations to anything that one might call sex. Heck, I was just a little kid. I didn't know enough about the world, about sex, or about my body to make the connection. So my enthusiasm for another trip down the slope in no way meant that I wanted to sniff or lick, kiss, squeeze or fondle, let alone penetrate or impregnate, my sled. And, I didn't end up with a luge fetish and spend my retirement savings on mail-order blow-up Flexible Flyer dolls to which I could whisper, "Rosebud" in the privacy of my bedroom. In fact, I soon became rather attracted to the opposite sex, dated numerous girls, and still have the hots for the beautiful then-15-year-old blonde I first saw six years later one block south from the site of my sledding experience. The vibrating sled merely produced stimulation to which my body automatically responded. So, relax. Even if you enjoyed the rectal exam a little bit (or a lot), it wouldn't mean that you were gay. I should note that even if you disliked the exam, it wouldn't mean that you were, therefore, not-gay, either.

Jokes about the rectal exam even show up in political humor, including this one by the master of sarcasm, Bill Maher, which includes a predictable swipe at his philosophical opponents. "New Rule: Stop calling it 'Obamacare.' It's not like Obama will be the doctor for your next prostate exam. That's just a common fantasy of Republican men" (*The Huffington Post* 2/5/2011).

Again, Dr. Rinaldi assured me: "Well, I don't really feel a lump, but the consistency of the tissue on the right side is just a little different. We'll need to have you see a urologist, but I don't think he'll find anything. Is there someone you'd like to see?"

The only urologist I knew had retired from his practice in our office building and became the county coroner. In that capacity he seemed to be fixated on asking questions about the masturbation activities of the deceased. I knew I did not want someone who had been associated with him.

"I usually use Rob Golden," said Dr. Rinaldi. "That's who I'd go to myself."

Good enough for me. I'd met Dr. Golden briefly at staff dinners of the Valley Hospital and Medical Center where I was a member of the "Associate Staff" as a psychologist, which meant that, while I couldn't admit or discharge patients (and didn't want to), I had privileges for visiting patients and being involved in their treatment while they were hospitalized. I scheduled an appointment with him for the next week.

The Prostate

Most books I've read about prostate cancer have included the designation "the size of a walnut," though I did see a couple of websites that referred to a "chestnut" or a "small plum" instead. Weary of reading about that freakin' walnut, I wrote a poem entitled "The Rancid Walnut," and thus conceived the title of this book.

THE RANCID WALNUT

The size of a walnut
all the books say;
this little gland provides
spasmodic delight
and a milky pool
for tiny swimmers destined

to spawn replications
of you and me.

Then like a rancid treat
stuck in the bottom
of your stocking
from Christmas
to Easter he hides
his amok-running cells
till the Periodic
Stimulation of Anxiety test
and some probing
of the ol' poopchute,
reveal that Mr. Prostate
is no longer your friend.

July 16, 2008[1]

The prostate encircles the urethra, just south of the bladder, directly in front of the rectum. This gland has an interesting structure, comprised of muscle and fibrous tissues intertwined in a dense mass. Without this little guy, our species may not have survived. The fluid produced by the prostate makes up most of the seminal fluid, provides nourishment to the sperm cells, and has a high pH (i.e., is a base). The alkaline nature of the fluid protects sperm by neutralizing the acidic environment of the vagina.

While it has been demonstrated that conception is possible without a prostate, it is still likely that the prostatic fluid provided a competitive advantage throughout evolutionary history. Sperm would be more likely to perish before they side-stroked their way up through Northern Fallopia without the protection of the prostatic fluid. Researchers now think the fluid also

---

[1] Previously published in the 2010 issue of *Blood and Thunder: Musings on the Art of Medicine.*

protects us from urinary tract infections that may damage reproductive structures. The ability to protect these critical structures is a characteristic that would probably increase the chances of passing on one's genes.

Whatever advantage the gland and its secretions provide, it's easy to see how such an organ could evolve to induce muscle contractions during ejaculation that propel the fluid and sperm cells out through the urethra. The contractions feel so good that the guy is eager to repeat the act—again, as soon as, and as often as, the opportunity arises.

But why would this gland evolve such susceptibility to cancer? After all, they say that nearly every guy will develop this disease if he lives long enough, and all too frequently it is fatal. If you think about it a bit more, though, the genetic susceptibility to cancer of the prostate would not be selected against.

Parents who passed on the genes that make a man more likely to develop prostate cancer would not have less breeding success than those who did not pass on such genes, since almost all prostate cancer is diagnosed in men over 40 years of age, with the vast majority of cases appearing when men are in their 50s and 60s or older. So, by the time a man first develops prostate cancer, let alone is killed by this slow-growing malady, he has pretty much finished procreating. At those ages, it is also likely that all of a man's children will be old enough that their survival is largely independent of whether or not the father is still living. Thus, even if prostate cancer killed every man while he was cutting into his 60th birthday cake, there would be no selective pressure against any set of genes that set us up for this disease.

The Biopsy

After another rectal exam at Dr. Golden's office, I heard more reassuring words. "I don't think we'll find anything, but we'd better do a biopsy." Dr. Golden described the biopsy something like this: "The procedure will involve me taking eight tissue samples from throughout your prostate through the wall of your rectum. I'll use an ultrasound contained in the probe to guide me. It will feel like a rubber band snapping inside your rectum." He prescribed hydrocodone for pain and Xanax® for anxiety, but said he thought he could probably get me through the procedure without the pain medication.

Now it is the morning of the test, and I have decided that even though I feel surprisingly calm, I'll take the Xanax®—my first psychoactive drug other than alcohol, nicotine (a dozen cigarettes and cigars in my younger years), and caffeine—just to make it easier. I don't notice any changes from the Xanax®. I wonder why my clients seemed to love it so much. Its effects on me are subtle, at best. I suppose I would have noticed a much greater effect if I were in the middle of a panic attack. I omit the hydrocodone.

Now I'm waiting in the examining room while Dr. Golden makes last-minute preparations for the biopsy. It dawns on me that I am fortunate not to be particularly modest. You see, I'm going to be bent over with my nether regions on full display, and this is not a one-person procedure. He's accompanied by an attractive blonde female assistant half my age. Many guys I know would be mortified, but I can count on one hand the times in my life that I have been embarrassed, and today isn't one of them.

I lean forward as instructed, and Dr. Golden inserts the trans-rectal ultrasound. The needle to extract the core samples is contained in the same apparatus. Now that I get a gander at the real thing, I realize that it looks sort of like a combination of the outer space ray-gun from the old Flash Gordon movies and a fire hose nozzle. Much as I loved Flash back in the 50s, I am a bit intimidated. It dawns on me that this device functions more as a rifle with night-vision scope than as an early space weapon, since it would soon be venturing into territory where the sun has yet to make an appearance.

Dr. Golden gives the signal and fires. It does feel sort of like a rubber band snapping in there, but it is more of a very deep ache in a place where you usually don't notice that sort of sensation. The unpleasantness is intense, but ebbs over a 10 to 15 second period. I'm glad I didn't bother with the pain medication. As I leave the exam room, I tell him, "That was less painful than the last 30 miles of a 100-mile ultramarathon, anyway."

On the way out, I see a framed photo on the wall showing Dr. Golden emerging from the mist of nearby Coeur d'Alene Lake at a New Year's Day Polar Bear Plunge. Soldiers say they respect an officer who's gone through the same ordeals he demands of them. I would not use my electronic training collar on my Chocolate Lab until I shocked myself with it a few times. I don't know whether or not Dr. Golden has undergone a prostate biopsy, but I think the swim gives him a pass. After swimming on the warmest summer afternoon, I shiver with cyanotic lips for several hours. My body fat level is currently well above the 7.9% measured when I was at the height of my marathon training, but I am still pretty thin at six feet tall and less than 160 pounds, so I'll take a biopsy-gun in the keister over a winter swim any day.

The waiting begins. I thought later about how patients in the past were sometimes not told that they had cancer—how often, even today, people will not utter the word, but stick with "the big C." I'd rather have it right out there to deal with. Thus, I appreciated Dr. Golden's style of breaking the bad news when he called.

"Steve, we have a problem with your biopsy. You have cancer."

Three little words we all dread. Describing his reaction to hearing those same words, my friend Mark said, "It seemed like the sun and earth stopped moving." That sounds about right. At least I found a poem in there.

THREE LITTLE WORDS

Bob Dylan said if you weren't busy
being born you were busy dying, and
as adults we know that's true,
but we never quite believe it as we do
when the physician says, "You have cancer."

I've always liked the sound
of "three little words",
but so far I've been blessed
with those that bathed me in affection.

I knew how to react to *those* words.

The rational response to the doctor's verdict
would be to activate myself,
to rush to complete each item
left waiting on my LIST,
to savor each sensation arising
from without or from within,
to be as present in each moment
as I sometimes am,
as present as
I only wish I could always be.

But the first response to loss is to retreat;
inertia clogs our behavior stream,
distraction clouds our focus,
and agitation mars appreciation of
experiences that are the stuff of life.

So, I'll muddle through,

accepting some dysthymic breaks,
alert for abject melancholy,
lest I spoil the unknown days ahead.
For our time here remains finite—
the Universe simply smacks some of us
with a few extra reminders.

January 25, 2008

Dr. Golden gave me a copy of the pathology report from my biopsy. Here is a shortened version:

PATHOLOGIC DIAGNOSIS;

A. Right prostate, needle core biopsies: Adenocarcinoma. Gleason score 6 (3+3), involving one of multiple biopsy cores, approximately 15% of specimen volume.

B. Left prostate, needle core biopsies: Adenocarcinoma. Gleason score 7 (3+4), involving two of multiple biopsy cores, approximately 15% of specimen volume.

The fusillade of strange words and numbers from this impersonal document hammered my eyeballs. Fortunately, I had read about some of the terms employed. The Gleason score measures the aggressiveness of the cancer. Each core sample from the biopsy is assigned a number from 1 to 5, depending on how regular and organized the cells are. Cells rated as 1 look perky and smooth, the picture of health. Cells rated 2, 3, and 4 are progressively more disorganized. By the time you get to a rating of 5, the cells vary greatly from each other in structure, many hardly recognizable as separate, distinct entities. The more disorganized the cells, the more likely an aggressive sort of cancer is involved.

The first rating refers the type of cell found to be most prevalent. The second number represents the second most common type of cell. These two ratings are added together to get the final score. Thus, a Gleason score of 7 could occur either with (3+4) or (4+3). Though both have the same total, it is much better to have a 7 (3+4), because that means that the largest number of cells have been graded as 3; whereas with a 7 (4+3), the largest number of cells have been graded 4, indicating a more aggressive cancer. Obviously, you want to see low numbers, especially in the first rating. My Gleason scores, 6 (3+3) and 7 (3+4), were in the high moderate range.

The information from the biopsy pathology report is combined with such things as your PSA, how fast your PSA has been changing (its velocity), and the way the tissues feel during the rectal exam. This process is called staging. Staging is a way to estimate the severity of your cancer. Based on my particulars, Dr. Golden said there was a 90 percent probability that the cancer was confined to the prostate. I won't detail all the levels of staging here. You can find this information in many other books (e.g., Walsh and Worthington 2007). What's important is that staging provides information for decisions about treatment. We'll look at the frustratingly complicated process of decision making in the next chapter.

So there it was: I had cancer. *Adenocarcinoma, in fact, whatever in the hell that is.* This thought sent me back to the books, where I learned that adenocarcinoma is a form of cancer that involves a malignant abnormality in the glandular cells. So that's what the hell it is, though such knowledge provides little useful information because nearly all prostate cancers are of that type.

I had joined a club whose membership is

burgeoning. According to the Johnson and Johnson®
2010 annual report, more than 900,000 new cases of
prostate cancer were diagnosed around the world in
2008. That same year, the number of men dying of this
disease increased by 16 percent to 258,000, compared
to the number only six years earlier. In the United
States, there were 217,730 new cases of prostate cancer
diagnosed in 2010, according to research reported in
The Journal of the National Cancer Institute (Farwell et
al. 2011). No wonder it seems as though every week
you hear about some friend who's just been diagnosed
with this disease.

There is something about the written word, isn't
there? That printed biopsy report slapped another red-
lettered stamp of reality on my disease. Clichés abound
when you try to put your reactions to such information
into words. It was just a few weeks before Christmas, and
now I needed to tell my two kids about my new condition.
It did seem surreal. Again, a predominant theme
reverberating through my head was: *This happens to other
guys, not to me.* Feeling sorry for oneself is a good thing
to counter, and counter quickly. How about another poem,
a crude one from some forgotten date that December?

CANCER DIAGNOSIS
Why me?
Why not you, Asshole?

December, 2007

Some who read that poem will be reminded of the
Denial stage of the grief process described by Elizabeth
Kubler-Ross in her classic book, *On Death and Dying*
(1969). That interpretation fits, for as I often told
psychotherapy clients, a question such as "Why me?" can

readily be translated to demanding statements such as, "This shouldn't be happening to me," "This isn't fair," and "The world must be different than it is." I have a Denial poem in a later section, but I also came up with some verse that suggests denial is a process that does not require us to be completely awake:

DON'T BLINK

sometimes when you awaken
there is the briefest of
treasured moments,
lasting, say,
less than a breath,
when you still live in
your childhood home,
your leg isn't in a cast,
Grandma is alive and
you don't have cancer.

April 6, 2009

Why Poetry?

You might be asking yourself, "What's poetry got to do with prostate cancer?" When I began this book, I recalled that the first poem I ever wrote was in 1992, when I was diagnosed with a serious cardiac arrhythmia called ventricular tachycardia. That poem is too long to be included here. However, it is interesting to note that to say I wrote the tachycardia poem is not really accurate. I had awakened at my son and daughter-in-law's condo, after driving to Seattle immediately following the diagnosis. I was stunned, to say the least. I had a Holter monitor affixed to my chest to record my heartbeats on a continuous basis. There was a notebook and pen on the nightstand and, without planning to, I picked up the pen and out came the poem. It wrote itself in about 20 minutes, finished, completed, and not edited or re-written. It was just there. I'd heard people claiming to have this experience of a piece of writing appearing unbidden, but had been skeptical. Now I knew what they were talking about.

It would be thirteen years before I wrote another poem. This time the writing was planned and deliberate. My friend, Bill Greene, had begun a writing group with local writing instructor Lisa Conger. They had obtained a grant from the National Poetry Therapy Association to conduct a group called "Write From The Heart," which invited health care professionals of all kinds to come together and write about important things in their lives.

Bill has a sneaky way of getting me involved in things, often by casually planting a seed well in advance ("You know, you'd do really well at that 50-mile mountain race in July.") This time he was more direct. He simply invited me to join the group. I was retired and had plenty of time, so I couldn't think of a good reason not to at least see what it was like. Everyone in this group of wonderful people seemed to be writing poetry, so I followed suit. I wrote about a variety of topics ranging from the death of my dog, to my grandmother's piano, meeting my wife, and long-distance running.

Licensed psychologists are required to take a certain number of hours of continuing professional education to maintain their licenses. Staying current and learning new skills is a good thing. On the other hand, the continuing education seminars are often mind-numbing, either because the material is so basic that you know you could conduct the workshop with half an hour to prepare, or because it is presented by some famous psychologist who is way too impressed with his or her own importance. Fortunately, every once in a while you hit a program that is useful. Sometime in the 1990s, I had attended a continuing professional education program that included a section on the benefits of writing about one's reactions to traumas and other difficult life events. Thomas Pennebaker, from the University of Texas at Austin, is the pioneer researcher in this area. One of the studies involved women with advanced breast cancer. The patients were divided into two groups. One group was told to go into a room and write for 20 minutes about their reactions to their disease. They were told that no one would read their writing; what they wrote would be discarded. The second group, as a control, was told to go into a room and write for 20 minutes about the items that were in their closet. That's it—that's the whole experiment.

The researchers sat back and waited, and checked on the groups later. It astounded me to hear that the members of the first group lived significantly longer than those of the second group. Many subsequent studies by Pennebaker (1997) and others have confirmed the health benefits of writing about difficult issues.

It seemed natural when I was given my prostate cancer diagnosis to write about it. I don't remember making a planned, conscious decision to do so. I just began. In our writing group, we have a prompt for each of our bi-weekly meetings. The prompt is usually a poem to which we are invited to react, either to a line, a phrase, or the general theme of the verse. Many times I did not write on topic, because I found myself writing about prostate cancer (and later about my heart surgery). Fortunately, the members of our group don't care what anyone else in the groups writes about. Everyone is always supportive and enthusiastic.

You will notice in footnotes after some of my poems that I have been able to get several of my poems about prostate cancer (as well as one about childhood polio) published in *Blood and Thunder: Musings in the Art of Medicine.* *Blood and Thunder* is an annual journal of art, photography, poetry, and prose related to health that is published by the University of Oklahoma College of Medicine. It was started in 2000 by a group of medical students. This publication is an example of training in medicine that includes study in the humanities.

Bill Greene retired from pediatrics in the summer of 2010. He has kept his hand in medicine since that time. He and Lisa now teach an elective course in which medical students write about their experiences, similar to our Write From The Heart group. I'm sure many people have dealt with at least one physician who they wish had been involved in such a humanizing endeavor.

A Project That Never Made It Off The Ground

This book arose out of a poetry project which I have at least temporarily abandoned. An idea came to me one day when I was out running, eight months or so into my recovery from surgery. I had already written six or eight poems about prostate cancer. *Why not do something to encourage others to do likewise? I'll invite men with prostate cancer and their families and friends to write about their experience.* I composed a letter about the therapeutic aspects of writing to all of the urologists in our area, to several of the top prostate surgeons around the country, and to a dozen or so family practitioners whom I knew locally. I requested that they encourage their patients to submit poetry about prostate cancer to me. I planned to compile these writings, add introductory and transitional material, and publish the result as a book.

Next, I contacted a delightful, talented young woman named Virginia De Leon, who wrote human interest features for *The Spokesman-Review.* We met for a couple of hours, and she talked with Karen about the way my cancer affected her. She arranged for Jesse Tinsley, a creative photographer, to add photos for the paper and a feature for their Internet publication. Virginia researched prostate cancer and wrote an article which included an invitation to others to submit material for my project, which I had titled *Prostatus Poetica*. [Our dear friend, John Brennan (1935-2010), an ex-Franciscan priest and thus a bit of a Latin scholar, informed me that I had the declensions wrong, that it should be either *Prostatus Poeticus or Prostata Poetica*. He acquiesced when I pointed out that my version sounded much more poetic. I wish he were still with us. He provided me with constructive, and even downright nasty, criticism in his endearingly Irish way.]

My enthusiasm for the poetry project was not matched by that of others. Neither Virginia's article nor my entreaties to physicians resulted in more than a handful of poems. Even directly contacting friends who'd had prostate cancer was to no avail. I suspected that a number of the guys who I thought might write were far enough along in their recovery that they did not want to revisit the experience. I'm sure there is a way to make such a project succeed, especially if there is contact with ongoing cancer support groups, but the results of my efforts were not enough to sustain my interest.

Maybe I would have gotten a better response if I had included this quote from Maya Angelou that appeared on the April 4, 2011, daily online post *The Writer's Almanac*. "There is no greater agony than bearing an untold story inside you." Anyone who has read her autobiographical work, *I Know Why the Caged Bird Sings,* can relate to the healing power of telling one's story.

My disappointment at the lack of response to my idea was mitigated by an unexpected response to the newspaper article. Several strangers sent emails wishing me well. I also began hearing from people whom I had not communicated with for three or four decades. In some ways, their response was disconcerting, since it seemed as though they were hurrying to speak to me before I died. Overall, though, it was uplifting, and I managed to maintain ongoing contact with some of these old friends.

Months later, I was again running along the river below our house, and out popped the idea for this book. If I wasn't very good at getting others to write, I'd incorporate my poems into a memoir focusing on my journey with prostate cancer.

I began with an outline in the fall of 2009. Without my abortive attempt at the *Prostatus Poetica* project, I doubt that I would have come up with the idea for *The Rancid Walnut*, so I'm glad that I at least tried to make the poetry project work. Perhaps people will read this book and write some poetry about their disease, or that of their loved ones, and I'll finally receive enough material to accomplish the original goal.

Emotions

Much of the focus of my poetry is on Emotions. Those Emotions, along with a Body that senses and performs Actions, Thoughts produced by the Brain, and, some would say, some sort of Spiritual component, is everything that we are. Each of these aspects of our being affects each of the others in a reciprocal manner. The following diagram is a variation of one created by my psychologist friend, Roger Harman, for a continuing education seminar. Roger's example was inspired by a diamond-shaped model used by Greenberger and Padesky (1995) to show the interactions between "mood," "behavior," "thoughts," and "physiology."

OUTSIDE WORLD (Past and Present)

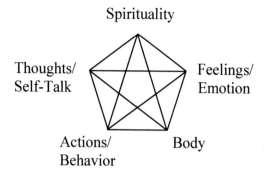

I recently found an example that illustrates the process summarized by this diagram in an unexpected place: an intriguing memoir written by A. J. Jacobs entitled *The Year of Living Biblically: One Man's Humble Quest to Follow the Bible as Literally as Possible* (2008). I vaguely recollect references to this book on the Internet that stressed pieces of scripture that almost no one would follow literally, such as Exodus 21:15, "Whoever strikes his father or his mother shall be put to death," and incomprehensible ones such as Numbers 19:2, about the importance of finding a perfect red cow.

I found that A. J.'s book is much more than a satire. It is a thoughtful and respectful recounting of his year-long exploration of Judeo-Christian theology, heavy stuff told with a light heart and a hefty dose of wry, self-deprecating humor. A worthwhile read.

In one passage, A. J. is wrestling with the issue of cleaning up his language, prompted by Ephesians 5:4: "Nor should there be obscenity, foolish talk or coarse joking, which are out of place." He describes missing a subway and then beginning to swear. When he substitutes "fudge" for the F-word, he notices that his anger recedes. Once again, *behavior shapes emotion* (emphasis mine).

Of course, feelings and thoughts also affect each other in reciprocal fashion and shape behavior, as when A. J. is so angry at missing the train that he yells at his wife or child after having the thought, *It's their fault. They always make me late.* I would guess that A. J. found, in turn, that his smile and diminished anger led him to milder internal bodily responses and fewer thoughts about the unfairness of the universe. And round and round it goes, in a loop that either exacerbates or has a calming effect on one's thinking, acting, and feeling.

An agnostic throughout the book, A. J. acts in ways that he would act if he, indeed, had faith. He is curious about the effect of such action on the spiritual dimension. At the end of the year, he still does not believe in a traditional biblical God. However, in the words of one of his spiritual advisers for the project, retired Lutheran minister Elton Richards, A. J. has become a "reverent agnostic." "I now believe that whether or not there's a God, there is such a thing as sacredness. Life is sacred. . . . There is something transcendent, beyond the everyday." (Jacobs 2008, p. 329) It seems that acting *as though* there is something to this spiritual stuff, has affected his spirituality.

Emotion has been discussed in, and has been the subject of, literature for ages. It is the stuff of romance, struggle, heroics, and meaning in life. Gripping writing grips because it evokes emotion in the reader. Emotion is also one of the sources of the profound hold that music has on us. However, emotion is not easy to study.

Throughout the history of psychology, researchers and theorists have most often defined emotion in terms of the private, internal experience of individuals, usually by referring to verbal reports of what is going on within their skin. Such reports are the easiest and most accessible indicators of private events, but the shortcomings of this approach are obvious. How can one know what other people are experiencing when they report feeling glad, sad, or mad? The experience is inside, private. No one else can see it, feel it, smell it, touch it, or taste it. What I mean when I report experiencing a particular feeling may be quite different from what you mean. The example of language development illuminates this problem. The unobservable, internal experience that a male toddler is having when he falls down may be very similar to that experienced by a female of the same age. However, the label that gets paired with the internal physical experience in naming that emotion may be very different. The internal experience does not come with a name automatically attached. If the little boy falls down and begins to cry, Mom has to guess what is going on inside of him, and then apply a label that matches her guess. Some moms might say, "Oh, don't be so angry." Some might query, "Oh, are you hurt?" Then, another time, Dad may be the one present, and he might command, "Hey, quit being a baby. You aren't hurt." Imagine this process with a wide variety of emotions that we learn to identify, and you see that it may often be difficult to identify what our own reactions are, and even more difficult to figure out what is going on with another person.

Finally, in 1954, psychologists Schacter and Singer (1962) conducted a classic experiment demonstrating that emotion requires more than just physiological arousal. I'll omit the details of their study, because I don't want to overload you with any more psychological research than necessary. Take my word for it: they clearly demonstrated that the emotion we experience requires both the physical reaction and the words—i.e., a cognitive label. The label reflects our interpretation of the arousal we are experiencing and the situation in which we find ourselves.

Men and Emotion

Learning about our feelings is complicated. Our social world is a major influence on our ability to recognize, understand, and manage our feelings. The social environment of men can lead them to be handicapped in their emotional lives. Not only are they frequently unable to experience and express their feelings, but they can have a hard time even identifying them in the first place. It's almost a cliché that we men often don't even know what we are feeling and have little patience with talk about such matters.

Individuals differ greatly in how aware they are of their emotional selves. At one extreme, some are classified with the high-falutin' term "alexithymia," which denotes an extreme lack of awareness of emotion. People who are alexithymic truly cannot tell you what they are experiencing inside. They miss out on an important source of information about the world and their reaction to it. It is easy to see how they would not do well in interpersonal relationships. In addition, a large-scale, 20-year study in Finland demonstrated that men with higher scores on a measure of alexithymia were more likely to die of cardiac disease (Tolmunen et al. 2010).

Men are especially likely to be punished for showing any sign of vulnerability, such as anxiety, depression, or feelings of helplessness. Think of John Wayne, whom people revere as a hero, when in fact he avoided military service during World War II and built up his career through a series of B movies in which he portrayed military heroes.

Celebrities play an important role as models for what's acceptable and what's not. In Wayne's 1971 movie *Big Jake,* his son (who, in fact, was Patrick Wayne, his son in real life) has gone off alone to try to catch some desperadoes who have kidnapped The Duke's grandchild.

His son is captured by the bad guys. I don't remember all of the details, but the life lesson from The Duke stands out. His son escapes and rides up to the good guys, dismounts, and walks up to his dad. Now what would most of us do? Think for a minute about how you, your spouse, your brother, or father would react in that situation.

What did John Wayne do? He hauled off and knocked his son off his feet with a roundhouse right.

What a guy. The only emotion our manly cowboy idol can display here is anger, and the only behavior he can show is aggression. My guess is that his reaction could be translated as, "I love you, and I was scared to death that something bad had happened to you," but wouldn't it have been nice to merely say so with words?

I believe the deficits that this kind of modeling and experience create in the emotional lives of men also prevent us from dealing with life-threatening illness as well as we could, if we possessed better emotional awareness and skill. In fact, it's that kind of learning that prevents so many of us from being "whole people."

People also vary greatly in how public they are when facing illness. Men as a group may be especially closed-mouthed when it comes to serious medical conditions, just as they are regarding sharing things such as the states of their marriages and the twists and turns of their emotional lives. One of my closest friends had a form of cancer, and I didn't learn about it until a year or so after his diagnosis. His treatment was brief, and all follow-ups have continued to show him cancer-free, for which I am grateful.

When he told me about his cancer, I was shocked and worried for him. At first, I was also disappointed that he hadn't told me sooner. It wasn't that I think there is one right way to be about the timing of sharing such information; when to do so and even whether or not to do so is clearly a personal decision. My disappointment was related to not getting the chance to be supportive of him when he was going through the process.

I'm at the other end of this sharing spectrum. For whatever reason, I am very open about the state of my health. I suppose some may find that either weird, or tiresome, or just plain narcissistic. As I will discuss later in the DECISION chapter, when I was devastated by the diagnosis of ventricular tachycardia, I published a poem and an explanatory essay in the local Road Runners Club newsletter, which would be read by several thousand people.

With prostate cancer, I have been open in speaking with friends and family. I also shared my experience through Virginia de Leon's newspaper article described earlier. Don't think I am telling you how much you should confide to others about your illness. We are all different. Be as private or public as you want to be. On the other hand, while I make no value judgment regarding this issue, as we will see, there is an advantage to actively dealing in some fashion with your emotions surrounding serious illness.

When men are unaware of or fail to acknowledge and deal with their emotions directly, they are more likely to cope by masking their feelings with drugs and alcohol. Or like Big Jake, they might find themselves swamped by the masculine default emotion of anger. Whether we refer to the process of dealing with cancer as grieving, or adapting, or coping, men will make their way through this journey more effectively if they are aware of their emotions than if they are not.

So far, I've talked about viewing emotion as a private experience, as a physical reaction, and as a verbal label attached to these internal events. In the last half-century or so, people have focused on more objective approaches to understanding this important aspect of life. Defining emotion has always been tricky. In graduate school, I was impressed by the completely objective, publicly identifiable, operational definition of emotion exemplified by the phenomenon of "conditioned suppression."

To demonstrate conditioned suppression, you teach an animal a behavior and measure that behavior over time under constant, controlled conditions, until you have a stable baseline of the action. For example, you reward a rat with pellets of food according to some schedule for pressing a bar. Maybe you provide the food after a number of responses that varies around some average. You continue doing so until the rat's behavior shows a consistent pattern over time. Then, while the behavior is ongoing, you introduce a tone followed by an electric shock. If you do this, you reliably see a dramatic change in the rat's behavior. Not only does it defecate and urinate (and give you the rodent version of The Bird, if you know how to observe carefully enough to detect it), but the ongoing behavior of pressing the bar will decline dramatically. Later, if you turn on the tone *without adding the shock*, the behavior will be suppressed as long as the tone is on, returning to the baseline pattern soon after you terminate the tone. Or, in more poetic human terms, from the earlier poem "Three Little Words":

> But the first response to loss is to retreat
> inertia clogs our behavior stream,
> distraction clouds our focus,
> and agitation mars appreciation of
> experiences that are the stuff of life.

I thought that the conditioned suppression paradigm was a cool operational definition of emotion the first time

I read about it, and I still do. Yes, it fails to capture much of the grandeur and allure we associate with the term "emotion," but it calls attention to a frequently overlooked part of emotional experience—namely, the disruption of ongoing behavior. Particularly with strong emotion, our actions do not flow as smoothly when we are experiencing the emotion as they do when we are feeling neutral.

Think about sports or academics. In sports, especially with performances that put a premium on motor coordination, excess emotion gets in the way. Take, for example, a golfer on the green who gets a case of the "yips," missing short putts when the stakes are high. Consider the basketball player who can hit 90 percent of her free throws in practice, but "short arms" them late in the game with the score tied.

Even if we haven't experienced it ourselves, we've all heard stories about people who are well prepared for a test who suddenly blank out in the examination room. Of course, we need a certain amount of arousal to complete any task. You can't pass the test if you don't give a damn or are half-asleep; you can't succeed in any aspect of sport without motivation and intensity. The relationship between amount of arousal and level of performance was summarized long ago by an inverted U-shaped curve given the name the "Yerkes-Dodson Law."

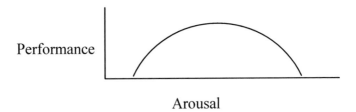

Arousal

At very low levels of arousal, performance is very poor. As arousal increases, performance improves up to a point, followed by a decline in performance to lower and lower levels as the arousal becomes more extreme. So, not only are some emotions like anxiety, panic, rage, and despair painful to experience, when they are excessive, they also can have disruptive effects that can spread throughout every facet of our lives. With prostate cancer, extreme, chronic emotional reactions can leave us focused on our disease, rather than on living a productive life.

Direct measurements of physiological reactions, such as those used in lie detector tests, have also been a way to access this complicated aspect of our lives. More recently, tools such as functional MRIs and PET scans are providing ever more refined views of brain events that mediate what we call emotion. The future of investigations using these new tools is bright.

Emotion, Psychological Stress, the Immune System and Cancer

As with heart disease and other serious illnesses, life style considerations such as dietary and exercise factors have been implicated as causes of cancer. There has also been a great deal of speculation about emotion and psychological stress as risk factors for these same diseases. The immune system is the most likely set of mechanisms through which emotion and stress would exert this influence. While the evidence for causative relationships between stress and the immune system is still tentative (see Segerstrom and Miller 2004, for a review), the field of psychoneuroimmunolgy has continued to progress over the last few decades.

The immune system is not a unitary entity. Instead, this term refers to an extremely complicated set of processes through which the body recognizes and fights foreign cells and organisms that invade it. At any given moment, we all have many damaged cells in our bodies. Sometimes these cells have been altered in such a way that they continue to reproduce at an extremely rapid rate, and without limits. Such out-of-control growth is the hallmark of cancer, and the cells are labeled malignant. The immune system is composed of a variety of mechanisms, such as natural killer cells and T-cytotoxic cells. These special cells attack and destroy malignant cells before they gain a foothold in the body. Malignant cells are classified as antigens and elicit this protective response of the immune system, just as do transplanted tissues which are also foreign to the body.

The National Cancer Institute (2008) published a Question and Answers document concerning psychological stress and cancer. Psychological stress was defined as ". . . the emotional and physiological factors experienced when an individual confronts a situation in which the demands go beyond their coping resources." Obviously, not all emotions are stress related. Feelings such as gratitude, relaxation, relief, and pride for a job well done have calming effects. These emotions are at the same time counters to stress and by-products of successful coping with difficult events. But reactions such as worry, anxiety and panic, and anger and rage, as well as hopelessness, despair, and depression, are directly tied to stressful life events.

The National Cancer Institute paper noted that the body's reaction of releasing increasing amounts of stress hormones such as adrenaline and cortisol in response to short-term stressors is helpful. Think about it—you have virtually the same anatomy and physiology as that which evolved long, long ago in a world where immediate, vigorous fight-or-flight reactions increased the chances of survival. The release of increased amounts of adrenaline into the blood stream, for example, quickly produced large increases in blood pressure and heart rate, allowing your great-great-great-great-great-great-great-great-great-great-great-great-great-great-grandpapa and grandmamma to react vigorously and avoid being lunch for some large, snaggle-toothed predator.

In our modern world, you rarely need such reactions. Threats to us today are rarely immediately physical. Yet we activate the same fight-or-flight system in response to chronically enduring factors such as job pressures, relationship difficulties, money worries, and concerns about the health and safety of our loved ones. When the stress response system that works so well for short-term threats stays activated for long periods of time, the immune system is suppressed and is less able to respond in a protective manner.

The National Cancer Institute paper noted a clear relationship between chronic stress and a variety of diseases, such as heart disease and depression. The links between stress and the immune system and the *development* of cancer are less clear. On the *Good Morning America* TV program, shock jock Don Imus stated with certainty that stress caused his recently diagnosed prostate cancer (Frias, Pereira and Ibanga, March 17, 2009). Of course, he is most famous for referring to members of the Rutgers University women's basketball team as "nappy-headed hos," so his pronouncements about medical science may not be particularly accurate.

In the same article, Dr. Otis Brawley, chief medical officer of the American Cancer Society strongly disagreed with Imus. "I am very confident we have no studies that show that stress is the sole cause of cancer, but stress can interfere with a person's ability to deal with cancer. The only risk that stress presents, in my experience and in scientific literature, is it sometimes makes it more difficult for someone to deal with the disease and actually get good therapy for it."

Support for the value of managing stress in terms of dealing with prostate cancer comes from a recent study reported in *Journal of Clinical Oncology*, which found that pre-surgical stress-management counseling with booster sessions following surgery led to lower levels of distress, anxiety and depression. A year later, the men who received stress-management training reported better physical functioning and improvements in quality of life than men given standard care (Cohen et al. 2011).

Both animal and human studies of cancer support the notion that stress increases the growth and spread of the disease once it is already present. Thus, if we already have cancer, our immune system function may very well help determine how fast the malignancy develops, and whether or not the cancer goes into remission. Twenty years ago, Sklar and Anisman (1981), working with tumors in mice, concluded that "[E]xacerbation of tumor growth is evident following acute exposure to uncontrollable but not controllable stress." In the Imus article, another oncologist, Dr. Mitchell Gaynor, made the strong statement that "[E]verything somebody can do as far as meditation, prayer, yoga, exercise—all those help prevent the recurrence of cancer."

I expect that more influences of stress on prostate cancer will be demonstrated in the future. An intriguing suggestion of the mechanism through which such effects occur was presented in a Wake Forest University Baptist Medical Center study in the online journal *ScienceDaily* (April 11, 2007). The researchers found that the stress hormone epinephrine causes changes in prostate and breast cancer cells that may help those cells survive.

Apparently, a protein called BAD (don't you love it), which is involved when cells die, is inactivated in cancer cells in the presence of epinephrine. Sounds like stress hormones could thus delay or prevent the death of cancer cells by interfering with one of the ways that the body destroys them.

These suggestions of links from stress to immune system suppression to cancer are tantalizing. Added to the evidence of the benefits of stress management for long-term recovery, they are enough to convince me to pay attention to keeping my immune system in tip-top condition. Even if the final word is that stress does not play a large part in the initiation or course of the disease, gaining skills to manage stress in your life can improve the quality of your days and help you to deal with whatever the disease throws your way. You have nothing to lose. If nothing else, you can live a more peaceful life.

Learning to monitor your stress levels before they become so extreme that they cause various symptoms, or even illness, is a first step. You will then be in a position to reduce stress levels by using relaxation methods and the cognitive-behavioral and self-management skills discussed in later sections of this book. There are also a variety of books available that can aid you in this regard, for example, *Managing Stress Before It Manages You* (Steinmetz et al.1980).

If these things called emotions have the potential to cause so much trouble, why do we have them in the first place? Emotions most likely evolved because they provided a survival advantage, as in the particular case of anxiety and panic and the resulting fight-or-flight, as discussed above. What kind of advantage? Emotions provide both information about the world and motivation to act. Fear warns us about danger and spurs us to escape or avoid it. Anger informs us about a trampling on our rights, a violation of our territory, whether such transgressions are physical or personal. We are, in turn, propelled forward to defend or attack. And sadness tells us we have lost something and helps us to retreat in order to heal. It is likely that in each of these cases, appropriate immune responses occur to maintain our bodily integrity, possibly in ways yet to be discovered by psychoneuroimmunologists.

It is maladaptive to be unaware of the signals our feelings provide. We miss the opportunity to act in ways that millions of years of evolution have proven to be useful. Thus, if you aren't very good at dealing with the emotional part of yourself, coping with prostate cancer will be more difficult. The private experience portion of your feelings will be more distressing. If you are unaware of your body's response to the stressors confronting you, you may not have a chance to come up with effective coping responses. Stress hormones, such as cortisol, which wear on the body, will be chronically elevated and may compromise your immune function when it might otherwise be able to gobble up any cancer cells hanging around in your prostate bed or beyond. Finally, your behavior may be affected in ways that interfere with living your life to the fullest. All the more reason to learn to do something about your emotions, rather than letting them control you.

Earlier, I noted the use of writing to cope with life's difficulties. Poetry can be a useful tool to begin gaining or regaining self-knowledge about what's going on inside of you. As the beloved American poet Robert Frost said, "People forget and poetry makes you remember what you didn't know you knew." (quoted on Suite101.com 2011)

You can become more aware of your feelings, acknowledge, respect, and honor them—and if appropriate, express them to others. Then get busy doing the things that allow you to live the life you want.

When my wise psychologist friend, Dennis Dyck, reviewed this section, he noted that, "How we manage our reactions to having a life-threatening illness, or even the process of dying, defines who we are and how we are remembered by those who know and care about us."

Here is one final thought about stress and cancer. I have spoken several times about my dog, Hershey. In the same continuing professional education workshop where I first heard about Pennebaker's work on writing about health and longevity, information was also presented concerning the benefits of having pets. It seems as though every week, there is an article about returning soldiers or autistic children being helped by working with horses.

Pennebaker stressed the value of dogs. He discussed research that showed elderly people who owned dogs outlived those who did not. It is tempting to speculate that reduced stress levels, social effects (though cross-species), and sense of purpose may be the mechanisms through which these benefits occur.

One possible confounding variable was noted, however. Dogs need to be walked several times per day. Maybe the benefit is due primarily to the increased activity level. After Karen was unable to continue her running due to plantar fasciitis and chronic Achilles tendonitis, she walked semi-regularly, averaging 3 to 4 miles, three times per week. During the five years we have had Hershey, she has walked at least 4 to 5 miles on 350 or more days per year. I am proud to report that over the last several months she has upped her mileage to 40 to 45 miles per week. Hershey is a happy boy.

Managing Emotions

How can a person hope to be able to manage these emotions when something as scary as cancer comes their way? The most helpful lessons I learned about this challenge occurred at a workshop in 1976. As an idealistic young man, I didn't want to be only a good listener who comforted people and helped them understand how their childhood experiences related to their current problems. I wanted to help them to make real changes in how they reacted, so that they could live more fulfilling lives.

I met my partner, Dick Groesbeck, in 1969 when we began teaching in the psychology department at Gonzaga University. In the fall of 1976, soon after we had started our private practice in psychology in the Spokane Valley, we received a brochure about a workshop in Seattle. Off we went for a weekend away, eager to learn new skills to help people who came to our office. We left the hotel room and mingled with a group of psychologists, psychiatrists and other therapists much senior to ourselves, all chowing down on donuts and coffee. The leader of the workshop was Albert Ellis, Ph.D., the Father of Rational Emotive Therapy.

From the beginning, I thought that Ellis was pretty obnoxious. I later read about his career, and his abrasiveness made more sense. He had been trained as a Freudian therapist, but when he used psychoanalytic techniques, he found that people were not getting better. He developed a therapy model based on what his patients were saying to themselves about the world, how they talked to themselves in their own heads. These ideas formed the basis of what was to become one of the most widely used and empirically-validated treatments for depression, anxiety and panic, post-traumatic stress disorder, and even notoriously difficult-to-treat personality disorders. Early on, though, the Freudians ruled the editorial boards of most journals, and Ellis was shut out. No one would publish his work.

Here was this outrageous guy up on the stage presenting these new techniques through clear, fascinating examples and witty, irreverent songs of his own creation. Though I found Ellis to be an unpleasant fellow, I was hooked on his ideas and began searching for more information, while Dick and I began implementing his techniques in our clinic.

Ellis called his methods Rational Emotive Therapy (RET). His techniques start with the assumption that our thoughts create our feelings. Ellis used the words of an ancient stoic philosopher, Epictetus, who said something to the effect that: "Men are disturbed not by things, but by the views they take of them." It's an A—B—C model where A, the Activating Event (what happens) is followed by B, the Belief (or Thoughts or Self-Talk or Interpretation of the Event), which is what causes C, the Emotional Consequence and resulting Behavior.

So, a girl turns you down for a date, and you tell yourself, *I'm worthless; no one will ever like me.* You then find yourself depressed. This reaction is likely to lead to isolation and withdrawal, rather than productive behavior such as pursuing a different woman. To remedy such an outcome, you can identify the irrational thoughts (B) and challenge them with more reasonable interpretations. For example, *Okay, she didn't want to go out with me. She's just one girl. I don't need to take it so personally. I can try again with someone else.* Now you may not be jumping for joy after the first girl rejects your invitation. After all, you did want to go out with her, and it's reasonable to be disappointed. However, that's a whole lot different from being depressed. And the resulting behavior is more likely to involve moving forward and finding other suitable partners, rather than staying mired in the muck.

Today, variations of these methods are referred to as Cognitive-Behavior Therapy (CBT), the term used by Aaron Beck (Beck et al. 1979.) Large, multi-site trials have given strong empirical support to the efficacy of CBT techniques in dealing with such problems as anxiety and depression. On February 15, 2011, our local newspaper, *The Spokesman-Review*, described a study in the latest *Annals of Internal Medicine* that demonstrated adding 20 sessions of CBT over a year's time for men who had had heart attacks led to a 45 percent reduction in subsequent heart attacks, as compared to a similar group not given CBT.

Karen and I recently found a new writer of suspense novels. In his recent work, *Intent to Kill*, James Grippando (2009) has someone suggest CBT as a treatment for the severe chronic insomnia the protagonist experiences after the hit-and-run death of his wife. The information about these techniques has even filtered down far enough that I recently saw a newspaper advice column recommend CBT by name to someone who had written for help. Now that's mainstream, Baby.

Throughout the remainder of the book, I'll provide examples of my irrational self-talk that generated emotions that complicated my own attempts to deal with prostate cancer. I'll also show you some of my attempts to help myself by challenging my "stinkin' thinkin'" by way of a more rational internal dialogue. First, obviously, is this earlier short poem:

CANCER DIAGNOSIS
Why me?
Why not you, Asshole?

Here, you see, the question *Why me?* is not really a question, but a demand. The question translates into, *This shouldn't happen to me; it's not fair.* A, the Activating Event, is the diagnosis of cancer; B, the Self-Talk, is the *Why me?* and C, the Emotion, is the resulting anger or despair, with its attendant self-defeating actions. A CBT therapist would first have me identify the irrational self-statements—in this instance, those related to fairness and demanding that the world be as I wish it to be. Next, I'd learn to challenge these ideas with more reasonable self-talk and then observe the resulting more adaptive emotions and behavior (*True, Steve, life isn't fair, but who ever said it was or should be? Life is what it is. Continuing to be sad or angry will only make things worse. Insisting that things have to be the way you want them to be is irrational and will only make you increasingly angry and depressed and prevent you from focusing on things you can, indeed, control. Get busy and deal with the situation in the best way you can.*) Of course, the second line of the poem provides its own succinct, though less diplomatic, counter-thought.

A first necessary step is to be aware of your self-talk, those exaggerated, irrational things you are saying to yourself. And we are often unaware that we are having these thoughts. They are the sorts of words and images that have been rumbling around in our heads for decades. Heavily practiced, they are as automatic as operating the clutch of a stick shift is for an experienced driver. Sometimes they are labeled "automatic thoughts," because they seem to appear out of nowhere. Because we often aren't aware of them, it takes some vigilance and effort to recognize that these powerful words or images are occurring inside our heads. Only after we have identified them can we challenge them with more reasonable ideas, and thus shift our moods and actions.

These automatic thoughts are often nearly unconscious. You don't usually sit down and say things like *Let's see—what does this mean? I have a diagnosis of prostate cancer, and so I will now die from it.* Well, sometimes you do, but often these sorts of thoughts are just there. They have become ingrained in your thinking, maybe even fading into the background as truncated representatives of the full thought. If you listen to yourself when you make a mistake, for example, you may detect in the background just a whisper of *Stupid* as the abbreviated self-condemnation *I'm so damn stupid. What an idiot. I always screw everything up.* You feel frightened or angry or depressed as a result of these self-statements and behave accordingly, even if you are not fully aware that they have occurred.

Don't get the idea that this CBT self-talk stuff is merely "positive thinking," or silly affirmations like those promoted by French psychologist, Emile Coue' (1857-1926), who had everyone walking around Europe saying, "Every day in every way, I'm getting better and better." While he should be commended for his early endorsement of the idea that our thoughts are critical to our mental health, his mantra is pure crap. We are complicated beings living under a difficult set of circumstances called The Human Condition. Every day, in some ways we are making progress, and in other ways we are sliding back and looping around. I doubt that it is helpful to lather your brain with that sort of Pablum®. It's more important to have a positive outlook, or a somewhat unrealistically positive outlook bolstered by a diligent countering of the overly pessimistic, depressogenic statements.

Several years ago, I created an outline to help my psychotherapy clients apply these strategies to manage their emotions and take control of their own behavior. I called it:

THE SEVEN Cs FOR COPING WITH MOOD PROBLEMS FROM A COGNITIVE-BEHAVIORAL APPROACH

The "Seven Seas" nautical pun was intended, because I saw this as a set of steps to guide each of us as we sail through the often-stormy waters that form our lives. Okay, corny as you might expect from me. I do like mnemonic aids. At least I didn't include a picture of a pirate. So here are my Seven Cs.

CATCH—Using your feelings or actions as a signal, remind yourself to observe your internal dialogue to catch your thoughts or "self-talk."

CALM—Allow yourself a few moments to take some relaxing breaths or to calm yourself by some other method.

CREATE—Out of your "self-talk," create a list of things you are telling yourself or images you are experiencing at this time.

CHALLENGE—Argue against or challenge any exaggerated, self-defeating thoughts that may be contributing to your depressed, anxious, or angry mood.

CHOOSE—Based on your more realistic thoughts, list your options for taking action and choose a set of behaviors that will move you further toward your goals.

COMMIT—Break those behaviors into small steps and commit yourself to following through by taking action.

CONGRATULATE—This work is not easy; you have put in significant effort to make these changes, so congratulate yourself for your efforts. When you do so, you are strengthening or reinforcing this set of behaviors so they will be more likely to be continued in the future.

This is a good time to note that with regard to the diagnosis of cancer, the medical community can only report probabilities to you, and that fact presents an excellent example of why it is so valuable to be aware of the things that you are telling yourself. A year or so after my surgery, one of my graduate school professors asked me if I had read Edmund Fantino's new book about his own prostate cancer. Dr. Fantino has taught and conducted research at the University of California, San Diego, for many decades. He is a Distinguished Professor of Psychology and Neurosciences who has been one of the top producers of cutting-edge research in Behavior Analysis. I immediately sent for a copy of *Behaving Well: Strategies for Celebrating Life in the Face of Illness* (2007) and quickly devoured this excellent piece of writing.

Though I have never met Fantino, I felt a connection to him, not only because of our shared disease, but also because we came from the same experimental analysis of behavior tradition in psychology. We also were both avid long-distance runners who loved the outdoors and were dedicated to our families. If there is only one book that you read along with *Dr. Patrick Walsh's Guide to Surviving Prostate Cancer* (Walsh and Worthington, 2007), which I discuss in the next chapter, it should be Fantino's *Behaving Well*.

I bring up Fantino's name at this point to highlight his description of some of his own irrational thinking connected with having prostate cancer. Fantino was rocked by his cancer diagnosis, and vastly more distressed when he woke up in the recovery room after his surgery and realized that not enough time had passed for the surgery to have been completed. After examining Fantino's pelvic lymph nodes, the surgeon had merely sewed him back up. The cancer had metastasized to the lymph nodes and was inoperable. Taking out the prostate after cancer has metastasized to the lymph nodes is generally viewed as the equivalent of wearing a condom after an egg has already been fertilized. "Day late and a dollar short," as Dad would say.

As Fantino and his wife began researching prostate cancer and its treatment, they read that he had a 29 percent chance of surviving for five years. He found himself focused on these gloomy statistics, which were especially devastating to a man with young children. Fortunately, it didn't take this brilliant researcher's mind long to remember that these data were averages. Some men with his level of disease lived longer, some for a shorter time. This more rational thinking jump-started his creative approach to living wholeheartedly for whatever period of life he had remaining. Last I heard, Fantino is still doing well, with over a quarter century of high quality life after his diagnosis.

I recently read an account by renowned evolutionary biologist Stephen J. Gould (1985) regarding his own profoundly bleak diagnosis of mesothelioma. As with Fantino, Gould's outlook improved as soon as he began thinking from the viewpoint of statistics. He countered his gloomy thoughts of imminent death by noting that the prediction he was given was based on a group, and that the outcomes of members of the group varied widely from one another. He did prove to be an "outlier," someone who survived much longer than nearly everyone else who had a similar diagnosis. Defying the dire forecast of averages, he thrived for another 20 years before dying of an unrelated cancer. Gould used his extra time to create a wealth of material to help us understand ourselves and our biological heritage. So don't despair if you are having difficulty controlling your irrational thoughts. Even brilliant scientists have to work at it.

In the FUTURE chapter, where I spend a great deal of time on methods of self-control, I'll present several additional methods for dealing with your disease and your life. While those strategies will provide additional help with your emotions, they will be more focused on teaching skills to manage your behavior.

Your Turn

Now, here is the difficult part about using any book that contains a self-help message. Most people will read the previous section and say to themselves something like, *Yes, that makes sense. Sure, I could do that. I'll bet that might work.* And then, as if they were reading a novel, they will proceed to the next section without actually applying the strategy in their own lives. I know; I've done it in the reading of dozens of self-help books. However, you will receive the greatest benefit from this book if you stop here and make a first attempt at working with these ideas.

Try it. Pick something distressing in your life, maybe related to prostate cancer if you or a loved one has the disease. Choose something that seems to generate more distressing emotion than you think is helpful to you. Write down a brief description of this as A, your Activating Event. Notice I said write it down. You will be tempted to do the exercise in your head, but for your first few tries, forcing yourself to put the words on paper will be more productive.

Next, examine your own thinking about this aspect of your life. What are the words (B) that come into your head when you are reminded of whatever it is that you have chosen? What emotion (C) results? Brainstorm to find other ways to talk to yourself about it. Write down alternative ways to think. For example, are you sure that what you are saying is 100 percent true? Are there exceptions? Could things turn out differently than you are predicting? What can you do to live a rewarding life, even if things do turn out as you fear?

Sometimes you may not be sure about what is bothering you, yet you know from how you feel or how you are acting that something is wrong, that your reaction seems to be hindering you. You can still use these methods to put yourself in a more favorable emotional state. Search for the self-talk. In the event you can't identify it, try this. Say to yourself: *I am acting as though I think that*_____. Fill in the blank—for example, *my life is over,* or *I'm completely helpless,* or *the world has to be as I demand that it should be.* Complete the exercise by countering those likely-present-but-hidden thoughts, and act in a way that is compatible with the new, more reasonable thoughts.

Now that you have practiced some with changing your self-talk, put everything I've discussed together. For example, here's what a Seven Cs exercise might look like. Let's assume that you have had a rising PSA, which is now at 7.0. Your doctor notices a lump during your rectal exam, and you have a biopsy that confirms that you have joined the millions of men who have cancer of the prostate gland. The urologist has given you some things to read, and you have talked to a radiation specialist. You have been bombarded with statistics about incontinence and erectile dysfunction that result from the different treatments. No fewer than ten people have called you with advice about what they think you should now do. It's 5:15 a.m. You've been up for half an hour, and you are at the kitchen table waiting for the coffee maker to finish brewing. The sun has just cleared the tallest trees on the horizon. Not a cloud to be seen. You watch the robins pulling up worms, harvesting their way across the lawn behind the path of the sprinkler. A grand summer morning full of promise. You are trying to read the newspaper. You find yourself rereading each short article and notice a nagging sense of discouragement. What are you thinking? Notice that there are a bunch of thoughts related to your prostate cancer swirling around in your head. Okay, great, you have now completed CATCH.

Put the paper down, sit with your hands loosely on your knees, close your eyes, listen to the birds calling, and take three deep breaths. Count slowly to four on the inhale, and count again on the exhale. Notice a muscle group somewhere in your body that seems tight or achy, and tighten it for a few seconds, then let it go. You've just used CALM to put yourself into a state more conducive to reasonable thought and action.

Let's CREATE that list of unreasonable thoughts now. You might discover self-statements such as, *Hopeless. I can't understand this stuff, can't figure out what to do. I'm going to die and not get to see my grandkids graduate from college and get married. Before that, I'll be wandering around with my limp dick flopping around in a smelly diaper.*

My List of Unreasonable Thoughts_____
_____
_____
_____
_____
_____.

Now, one by one, CHALLENGE those exaggerated, stress-inducing words. For example: *Come on, nobody has said anything about hopeless. Nobody suggested I'd croak soon. Each of the doctors spoke optimistically about my prognosis. I need to remember that Doug, and Mike, and Larry all had the surgery several years back and seem to be living happy lives. And didn't that book say that only 2 percent of men end up incontinent in the long run, and anywhere from 60 to 80 percent still get erections? It's fine to feel sad and worried. After all, this is cancer.*

My List of Rational Thoughts to Challenge Self-Defeating Thoughts _____

_____

_____

_____

_____

_____.

You might follow up with something like: *But I'd better CHOOSE to quit moping around. I'm going to continue to read the prostate cancer books for a half-hour each day and talk with people to help me decide what to do. In the meantime, I'm going to get myself moving.*

Behaviors I Choose to Help Me Move Forward

_____

_____

_____

_____

_____.

I'll walk the dog right now and promise myself to COMMIT to ten minutes over coffee each morning to write down a plan for doing things that I enjoy each day.

My Method of Commitment_____

_____

_____

_____

_____.

I'll also remember that it is not easy to follow through on these self-change methods, so I'll CONGRATULATE myself for doing this Seven C's exercise to help me move forward.

My Congratulations to Myself_____

_____

_____

_____.

If you wish to become a bit more sophisticated with these methods, you would do well to learn about various types of cognitive errors that we often make. You will find that most, if not all, of your distressing thoughts fall under one of the categories, such as those listed by David Burns in his wildly successful self-help book for dealing with depression, titled *Feeling Good: The New Mood Therapy* (1980). Rather than detail each of these types of thinking, I refer you to Burns to read about self-defeating thinking patterns such as: Overgeneralization (*I went off my diet; I never accomplish anything*), Labeling (*I'm an idiot*), Jumping to Conclusions (*My wife is in a bad mood; I must have done something wrong*), and Emotional Reasoning (*I get frightened whenever I think about my cancer; therefore, it must be a really advanced disease that will kill me quickly*).

There are other effective ways to deal with stress and emotional overreactions. I contemplated laying out the entire stress-management model that Dick Groesbeck and I constructed in the 1980s. I decided, however, that including sufficient detail to do that model justice would require more space than was warranted for this book. Maybe I can later motivate myself to make that model the basis of a separate book.

I previously mentioned the Steinmetz et al. stress-management book. For our purposes here, I think adding some of the mindfulness techniques related to meditation that can be found, for example, in the audio book *Mindfulness for Beginners* by Jon Kabat-Zinn (2006) or his book *Coming to Our Senses: Healing Ourselves* (2007), along with the use of the self-management skills outlined in the later FUTURE chapter, will suffice. Also I was pleased recently to run across *Cognitive-Behavioral Stress Management for Prostate Cancer Recovery*, a facilitator's guide and workbook for implementing a multi-week group program for men who have had prostatectomies (Penedo, Antoni and Schneiderman 2008). These two books are advertised as free downloads. However, when I tried to access them, I was asked for a $4.95 membership fee from the downloader. Still a good price, and I may sign up later. Don't think you to be in a group to use such material. I have had psychotherapy clients who worked individually with similar workbooks for anxiety, depression and panic disorder with good results.

I hope that as I continue with the story of my journey, I can help you to use these techniques from science, literature, and poetry to live effectively with your disease.

2

DECISION

Making a decision about which treatment path to follow when a man has prostate cancer is more difficult than the decision with most other diseases. Of course, this may not be true for everyone, especially for those who do not ask a lot of questions. If the urologist consulted makes a straight-forward recommendation of one treatment versus another, many men will merely follow along with the option suggested. I have spoken with some men for whom that has been the case.

I find it fascinating how greatly people differ in terms of curiosity about their health and health problems. Our dad was a very bright guy. With only a high school education, he began working for Continental Baking Company, running a bread-wrapping machine in Salt Lake City in the 1930s. Over the years he worked his way up to Regional Manager, responsible for the sales of Wonder Bread and Hostess Cake products such as Twinkies®, Cupcakes, Ho-Ho's®, SnoBalls® and Ding-Dongs® throughout Washington, Oregon, Utah, Idaho, and northern California. Wonder Bread products were revered in our household. One of our family stories Mom told was about me at age five or six, refusing to eat lunch at my Aunt Betty's house when she made the sandwiches with Table Queen Bread.

Dad's ability to earn similar loyalty from his employees was brought home to me repeatedly when men would come up on the street years after he had left town, to tell me that he was the best boss they ever had. He was a creative thinker. I remember his talking about cutting the bread into wider slices. People bought bread by the loaf and ate it by the slice, so if he produced a loaf with fewer slices, they used it up more quickly, and returned for another one. He also invented Tiger Tails®, the Twinkies® wrapped with the sweet pink coconut stuff, rather like barber poles. How cool is that? Yet despite his creativity, social astuteness, and sharp mind, Dad showed little interest in learning about his heart and vascular problems, his prostate cancer, or his Parkinson's disease. While I never talked with him about this issue, I think that the strategy worked for him, though I think he might have made some better lifestyle choices if he would have become more informed.

I'm just the opposite—I want to know everything I can about what is wrong with me, how the particular part of the body in question works, why it gets screwed up, and what my options are. Part of the difference between people on this issue may relate to the degree of comfort with reading scientifically-oriented material. Some people never did like science class, and have little, if any, experience reading in anatomy, physiology, or medicine.

Maybe Dad didn't think he could understand the medical information, or maybe it was just that he was from a generation that habitually accepted what the doctor told them (while not necessarily complying with the specific lifestyle recommendations that the doctor might have made). Or maybe, like many people, he found it less scary to remain unaware. Possibly it was just more comforting to avoid thinking about his health problems. While it can be a problem when it keeps us from taking steps to improve our lot, denial is certainly one technique that can help us cope with life's difficulties.

On the other hand, I've always had considerable interest in science, particularly biology. One of my favorite undergraduate courses was introduction to biology. While that was the only biology course I took as an undergraduate, I did take several courses in physiological psychology. At Gonzaga University, Dick Groesbeck and I taught a course in animal behavior together. Later we teamed with a biology professor and another psychology professor in an inter-disciplinary course we called "Contemporary Issues in Human Biology." In graduate school at Utah State University, I created my own minor, Wildlife Science/Ecology, by taking a selection of undergraduate and graduate courses in the Biology Department. There was no listing in the university catalog for an official minor under the heading of "Wildlife Science/Ecology." One of the advantages of being a bit older as a graduate student and having some college teaching experience was that I had the chutzpah to choose those courses that interested me and inform my committee that they comprised my minor.

In the end, sort of through the backdoor, including my own independent reading and getting mini-lectures on medicine, anatomy, and physiology on thousands of miles of runs with my pediatrician friend Bill Greene, I had studied a fair amount of biology before I was diagnosed with prostate cancer. Sometimes I think I would have been happier if I had majored in biology, but that's probably just another example of "grass-is-greener-what-if" musing of an old man.

When I was diagnosed with my arrhythmia in 1992, at the age of 38, I bombarded my cardiologist, Dr. Harold Goldberg, with requests for material about ventricular tachycardia. Following the diagnosis and the initial angiogram to rule out coronary artery disease, I had a second session in the catheter lab, where it was clear that Dr. Goldberg was not going to be able to ablate (burn away with radio waves) the unruly cells and cure me of the arrhythmia. He then told me he was prescribing Tenormin® (generic name atenolol) to control the dangerous rhythm. Atenolol is a widely used, but often hated, beta-blocker drug, due to its effect of reducing the rate and intensity of the heartbeat to such an extent that people find it difficult to do much physically while on the drug. I told him that I first wanted some evidence that this was a necessary path to follow with people like me, who were extremely fit and able to run 100-mile ultramarathons. Dr. Goldberg probably thought I was a bit of a pest, for I am quite certain that nearly all of his patients merely say "okay" when he prescribes a treatment regimen. He did his best, though, providing me with a stack of articles from medical journals dealing with my problem. None, however, addressed the issue of extreme fitness. I read more on my own and, in the end, complied with his suggestions. As expected, my ability to run was seriously compromised by this drug. Within a few months, I switched to sotalol, a new beta-blocker with specific anti-arrhythmic properties but with fewer of the bothersome side-effects of atenolol. Most importantly, sotalol interfered with my running performance much less than had atenolol, while still controlling my arrhythmia.

Over time, Dr. Goldberg came around with regard to my running. After all, he's a scientist. I showed repeatedly that, wired up for an exercise EKG, I could push myself to the point of dry heaves on the treadmill and still remain in a normal rhythm while on sotalol. He had the data. In place of his original suggestion that I limit my running to easy five-mile jogs, he routinely asked about my competitive running.

I followed a similar strategy of information gathering with prostate cancer. In fact, because no one can tell you which treatment is best, I became immersed in study of the disease. Dr. Golden had given Karen and me *Dr. Patrick Walsh's Guide to Surviving Prostate Cancer* (2001), along with a book titled *100 Questions about Prostate Cancer* by Ellsworth, Heaney and Gill (2003). I read these, and then found Walsh and Worthington's revised and updated (2007) edition and read that, too. Of course, one of the great things about the Internet is that I was also able to read a wide variety of articles that I found there.

The Importance of Taking Control

Just as with the positioning of the hide-a-bed on the morning of my surgery, I think that all this researching was related to a desire to feel in control. Being able to affect the world, to modify things of a physical nature as well as influence aspects of our social environment, is essential for our survival. We see the baby flailing randomly in her crib. When she strikes a mobile hanging above her, she is more likely to repeat the action, because it changes her world. It doesn't take long for her to learn a wide variety of behaviors that result in attention from the adults around her. She quickly gains a great deal of control over her social world. Thus begins a life of gaining increasing amount of control over the things and events that are keys to survival.

Non-human animals also must affect their world. They need to catch prey, find food and water and shelter, and they must mate if their kind is going to continue to exist. It has been clearly demonstrated that they not only exhibit behaviors that control the world, but that they also prefer situations in which they have choices when it comes to how they do so. For example, Voss and Homzie (1970) found that rats preferred finding their food by taking a path where they had two choices of routes, rather than taking a second path that only had a single route. A.

C. Catania (1975) extended this finding to pigeons. He allowed the birds to choose between a situation where they had only one key (a green one) they could peck to obtain food, versus another situation where they had a choice between pecking a blue or an amber key. No matter which key they chose, they received the same amount of food. The only difference was that in the first condition, they had just one way to earn the food, and in the second condition, they had the opportunity to choose one key over the other. The birds showed a clear preference for the situation in which they had a free choice. Even rats and pigeons will choose to choose if given the opportunity, at least under some circumstances.

I don't want to overwhelm you with more research studies, so take it from me that there are also studies showing that animals prefer situations where the world is predictable, as compared to situations where it is not. Thus, my seeking information is firmly grounded in my biological heritage.

Okay, animals like to be able to predict events, and they prefer being able to have choices in their lives. What about being able to control life events? Remember the study by Sklar and Anisman, in which tumors in mice grew faster when the animals were exposed to uncontrollable stress? Even a mouse with cancer benefits from being able to affect his world. But does taking control actually make a difference for us humans? Does it just make people happier? Does it also affect their health, their actions related to their health, and their actual health outcomes?

An example with humans astounded me when I first heard about it. If you are like me, one of the things that makes the notion of living in a nursing home distasteful is the resulting loss of control over so many aspects of daily existence. How does such a loss of control affect people, and what can these facilities do to make things better? Rodin and

Langer (1997) addressed these questions in a paper with the lofty scientific journal title of "Long-term Effects of a Control-relevant Intervention with the Institutionalized Aged." Nursing home residents were divided into two groups. One group was given a speech focusing on the idea that they had considerable responsibility for their own lives. They also were given the choice of which night they wished to attend the weekly movie, and were given a house plant for which they were completely responsible. The second group was given a speech that did not refer to responsibility, were told which night they would go to the movie, and were given a house plant that would be cared for by the nurses. That's the whole experiment. After a year and a half, the people in the individual responsibility group, who had been given more control over their lives, were happier and more active.

Now that is wonderful, and maybe mildly surprising. However, the result that blew me away was that only15 percent of these people had died after 18 months, while 30 percent of the people in the control group had died. Being able to affect the world may be a matter of life and death.

In *Behaving Well*, Fantino (2007) cited some of these same and related studies that emphasized the value of taking control. If the reader takes only one message from his book, it should be that when life-threatening illness strikes, it is important to take control, and that there is always something which we can control. Fantino's book is an argument against passivity. *Behaving Well* reminded me to focus on the importance of taking an active part regarding my illness, to take control of everything I could.

Of course, as I reflected on my reactions to this disease, I knew that taking control had been an important part of my strategy from the beginning. Don't forget that stupid hide-a-bed. True, there is a limit to how much we have to say about events outside of ourselves, including the behavior of others. And certainly, despite our best efforts, our disease may advance, even to the point at which it kills us.

I heartily recommend that you read *Anatomy of an Illness as Perceived by the Patient* (1979) by Norman Cousins, which documents his use of a positive attitude and humor to cope with a serious illness. In the end, each of us can emulate people like Cousins and Fantino by taking steps to alter the way we view the world, change the internal words we use to talk to ourselves, and exert control over the actions through which we live each moment of our existence.

Feeling helpless is one of the worst experiences I've ever had. Maybe that relates to the search for control that I have spent so much time discussing. Four decades ago, Martin E. P. Seligman, who later was president of the American Psychological Association, coined the term "Learned Helplessness" and published a book with that title (Seligman 1975). In a series of experiments, he showed that when dogs were put in a situation where they experienced unavoidable electric shocks, they later would take no action to escape the shock in a different situation, even when the shock was made escapable and avoidable. All they had to do in the new situation was jump over a small barrier to escape. Normally, dogs easily learn to perform this escape and also to avoid the aversive stimulus, if they are given a warning beforehand that it is coming. Instead, after being exposed to a world in which they had no control over extremely unpleasant events, the dogs in these studies gave up. They would lie passively and take the shock. Thus, they had learned to be helpless, even in situations where objectively they were not.

Seligman cited a variety of studies that showed this phenomenon also occurs in man. Learned Helplessness increases anxiety and affects our ability to think and problem-solve. In turn, having control decreases interfering emotions such as anxiety, and improves our ability to problem-solve. Work in this area confirms that we want to find predictability in our lives and to be able to exert control. In fact, the control need not even be real. Just believing that we have some control lessens anxiety.

Learned Helplessness became an experimental model of depression. I view my efforts toward garnering a sense of control related to prostate cancer as an anti-depressive technique. Having some sense of control counters the sense of helplessness that otherwise messes up my mood and gets in the way of going about enjoying my days.

Information and Control: How Much Is Enough?

I have described the substantial effort that I made to educate myself about prostate cancer and its treatment. I found this research to be helpful. However, even if one is comfortable reading scientific/medical material and is curious about his disease, there may be limits to how much information a person wishes to confront. I don't think it is unusual to get to a point where you are squeamish about the information.

When I was wading through the literature about prostate cancer, I found an Internet site that included a great deal of detail about the radical retropubic prostatectomy that I eventually had performed. I had read the description of the procedure in Walsh's book and studied his black and white line drawings of the way in which the anatomy was altered during surgery. It was not easy for me to view these drawings. I found they frequently caused near-lightheadedness and the contraction of various sphincters, some of which I may not even have known that I possessed until that time. The online site included a set of videos, in living color, of a prostatectomy. My index finger lingered on the top of the left button on my mouse. I started to click. I paused. I started again to click. *Naw. I'll pass.* I just couldn't do it. I had all the information I needed.

I'm not alone in choosing to place a limit on the amount of information I gather in such situations. Let me give you some examples that show even doctors sometimes make similar choices in the face of illness.

Bill Greene and I have run together on a regular basis for thirty years. He is the picture of health and fitness: non-smoker, vegetarian, very lean, extremely active (always among the top placers in his age group in long-distance races, easily beating the vast majority of people in younger age groups), involved in meaningful work which he enjoys, and he is surrounded by a large number of family members and friends who love him. Bill and I have run thousands of miles together on streets, roads, and in the mountains for distances of up to 62 miles. I paced him the last 38 miles when he completed the Western States 100 Mile Endurance Run from Squaw Valley to Auburn, California.

Join Bill and me in early September, 2009, while we are training for the Le Grizz 50 Mile Ultramarathon in northwest Montana. Friday morning, we had driven up to the summit of Mt. Spokane and spent five hours running on roads and cross-country ski trails. Though I always carry my cell phone when I run, I noted to myself later that on this run, we ventured beyond cell phone coverage due to the shadow of the mountain. We had an enjoyable day. Now it is Sunday morning, and our plan is to take an easy seven-mile run on the Centennial Trail along the Spokane River below my house.

At our turnaround point, we pick up the pace a bit, but are not pushing to the point at which we have even begun to breathe hard. All of a sudden Bill stops, crouches down at the side of the trail, and begins taking his pulse. I look down at the receiver unit of his training heart monitor and notice that it reads 10:40. The monitor is in the Time of Day mode, but the little heart symbol is jack-hammering away like the heels of a flamenco dancer. "Turn it to the Heart Monitor mode, Bill."

When he pushes the button and the dial reads 191, I know something is wrong. He remains in a semi-squat, head down. Within a minute, the monitor jumps back to 74. The arrhythmia has converted to a normal rhythm. He stands up. "Let's just walk home, Bill." As we begin to walk, he grumbles, "I've been standing too close to you all these years." We both are thinking that he has developed a tachycardia similar to mine, and that he will be going in for a stress EKG in a few days. After walking for a while, he says, "Let's just go ahead and run back easily." We do.

It isn't until the next day—when he calls me from the hospital to tell me that he's had a heart attack and is going in for an angiogram—that my stomach flip-flops at what might have happened when we blithely ran home after his event. The possibility that his trouble could have occurred up on Mount Spokane makes me shake in my boots. Later that week, he has quadruple-bypass surgery.

Bill is a perfect example of how humans are both vulnerable, even though we might follow a healthy lifestyle, and resilient when our health is compromised. Eight months after his surgery, Bill placed fifth in our very competitive age group at the Lilac Bloomsday 12 Km run, and not long after the first anniversary of his surgery, he completed a marathon at a 9-minute per mile pace, an excellent performance for any 66 year-old. How's that for a recovery?

As I spent time with Bill during his recovery, I realized that he, too, limited the amount of detail he was exposed to concerning his surgery. Of course there was not much time to study before the surgery, since the procedure was completed a few days after his first symptom. However, even during the months following his bypass, he did not delve into all the details of what when on when he was in the operating room. Wisely, he did an extensive review of the best recommendations for preventing atherosclerotic disease in the future, and he has done an admirable job of following such guidelines.

I was discussing the issue of how much a person wants to know about his health problems with another friend, who is a retired orthopedic surgeon. He described his own experience with surgery to remove polyps from his nasal passages. "They wanted to tell me about the procedure. I had done the research I needed to do about risk factors and had used enough scopes on people. I knew they were going up into my turbinates. That was enough detail. I said, 'Just get rid of my polyps.' I didn't want to know."

E. Fuller Torrey is another physician who had prostate cancer. In his book, *Surviving Prostate Cancer* (2006), he describes a scene in which the pathologists called him over to see his biopsy under the microscope. He lingered there only briefly before leaving with the thought that what was an interesting intellectual exercise for them, was a possible death sentence for him.

Emotional Reactions to Decision-Making

In the midst of the decision-making process, I found myself dealing with a variety of emotional issues. Not surprisingly, fear was a big one. I also found myself both angry and sad. I had been a psychologist in private practice for 28 years, so I have had extensive practice in helping people deal with such phenomena. This kind of experience did not guarantee that I would have smooth sailing through this emotional sea. As with physicians who continue to smoke cigarettes, I found it sometimes easier to give than to follow good advice.

Karen and I have always followed a healthy lifestyle. The first time my attention was captured by anything in particular one could do for better health was in my freshman year at the College of San Mateo. My family, like most in America, had always viewed meat—especially beef, and even more especially beef steak—as the center of the very best eating experience. Hell, Grandpa Bren had run his own meat market in Salt Lake City for most of his working life. When Dad was away in the Navy during World War II, Mom, and Aunt Eva and Uncle John, and we kids always had beef on the table. Rationing didn't get in the way for Grandpa Bren, who always had a bit of a shady side to him. It sounds like a cliché, but he really did have his thumb on the scale while he distracted the ladies with his "bedroom eyes," to use Mom's phrase. The value of meat in Karen's family was shown when she asked her dad for money to buy a new dress. He said yes, but told her the family would just have to eat beans for the next few weeks.

My first semester at the College of San Mateo found me in a course in health that was required for the Associate of Arts degree. The course was taught by a diminutive, arrogant physician from the community. I didn't particularly like him. Maybe it was because I got a B in the class when I knew the material backwards and forwards. Or maybe it was because he spouted off some ridiculous opinions disguised as facts.

For example, one day he stated that there was no such phenomenon as the female orgasm. Women were just confused by urinary tract irritation, he said. That must have been helpful information to his young charges, especially since no one challenged him. Not a word! I hadn't thought of that for years. Can you imagine the reaction of today's coed to such nonsense? But I digress—sex talk does that to me.

A few years later, I heard that this same physician had died of a brain tumor, so maybe I should cut him some slack. To be fair, I must note that he did provide other information that I found both useful and believable. His lectures about coronary artery disease were backed up by the text and, thus, seemed like more than just his opinion. He described dramatic atherosclerosis in the autopsies of young American soldiers killed in battle. Japanese soldiers, with a diet that was not heavy on meat, showed no such narrowing of their coronary vessels. I was impressed by this information, especially the pictures of cross sections of coronary arteries in members from the two groups. When Karen and I married the next year, we began to limit the amount of meat we ate. As the years progressed, we came gradually closer to a vegetarian diet.

This tale of families and views of meat is important when I consider some of my reactions to both my cardiac issues and my prostate cancer. Just as with many of my psychotherapy clients, I found myself (and the use of past tense here is probably disingenuous) repeatedly complaining in my head that the world was unfair and demanding that it should be different. After all, I had led a healthy lifestyle. I had done what I was supposed to do, so why the hell should I get prostate cancer?

Check out one more poem, chunks of which kicked around in my head for years before finding their way onto paper. I suppose it was also influenced by Bill's having a heart attack, despite his having done just about everything a person could do to promote cardiac health. The major risk factor of genetic predisposition may have overwhelmed all the proactive actions that he had followed. His dad died of a heart attack at the age of 62. The only controllable risk factors that I have been able to discern in him are a history of sleep apnea and a substantial red wine deficiency. This poem relates to prevention, but also begs to be analyzed from the framework of the self-talk of CBT. Am I making an irrational demand that the world must be the way I want it to be? Or can it be read as showing some degree of acceptance of the reality that confronts me? Or both?

WHINY LIFESTYLE LAMENT

nothing is fair in terms of health
the time you die's beyond your wealth

be active for your every day
no smokes save first in bales of hay
eight hours soft slumber for your night
of red meat there's not e'en a bite
munch green and red, orange and yellow
perfect yoga till you're mellow
relax, wind down, stay cool and calm
immersed in ever-prayerful balm
despite these plans, this style of life
disease still slips through like a knife
your neighbor does advice ignore
sofa-bound, movement just a bore
brown stain lies upon his finger
spot on lung will never linger
consumes without desire's restraint
watchful regimen all too quaint
see him skate with no malady
train-wreck near were he you or me
and never think your rice and beans
will ever trump his lucky genes

nothing is fair in terms of health
the time you die's beyond your wealth

February 27, 2011[2]

Okay, I didn't deserve to have cancer. But whoever said things were fair, or that deserving or not deserving had anything to do with it? Maybe it's time to repeat the use of the CBT methods. Again, I admit to being more

---

[2] Previously published in the 2010 edition of *Blood and Thunder: Musings on the Art of Medicine.*

proficient at doing this sort of analysis and challenging unrealistic self-talk with others than I am with myself.

In his book, Patrick Walsh noted that the relationship between physical activity and prostate cancer remains unclear. He cited one study that showed a lower incidence of prostate cancer in older men who were more active than their more sedentary counterparts. However, he also described a discussion with Dr. Kenneth Cooper of *Aerobics* fame about what seems to be increased level of the disease in young, lean marathon runners. Cooper blames free radicals, which are increased by extreme exercise, and are also intimately involved in the oxidative processes that cause cancer. He recommended that endurance athletes increase consumption of antioxidants.

For years, I trained and raced extremely hard without much thought about antioxidants or prostate cancer. Two of my ultrarunning friends, who joined me in the Chief 10 Bears Club for those who logged 20 completions of the Le Grizz 50 Mile Ultramarathon, have also been treated for prostate cancer in the last few years. That means that 50 percent of the "Chiefs" have had the disease. (Well, 3/7, but Mary Ann "Coyote Woman" Clute doesn't count, for the obvious reason.) We are all in the prime age-range for prostate cancer, but 50 percent seems to be an elevated number. Is this just a statistical artifact, or is excessive exercise a factor? Should I have chosen not to run ultras? Been less competitive? Consumed more antioxidants? So, here is another example of nutty internal dialogue I have noticed.

At several points, I became aware that my thoughts had turned into blaming ones such as, *I wonder what I did to cause this problem. I must have run excessively and generated a humongous number of free radicals. By pushing myself, being so competitive and pursuing those challenges like 50 and 100 mile runs, I brought this on myself. It's my fault.* Fantino (2007) reported a similar pattern in his own thinking when he found that his cancer had metastasized: *"Somehow I felt it was my fault and I apologized to Stephanie. I was emotionally stunned and kept thinking of how I had let my family down."* (p. 9)

The following poem is an example of challenging such irrational thoughts.

ASSIGNING BLAME

In Samuel Butler's
Erewhon, citizens
were blamed for
their own ill health.

Moderns claim
free radicals from
excess exercise
promote prostate cancer.

I ran 60 ultramarathons
and had a prostatectomy.

It's hard to lump myself
with lung-cancerous
smokers,
fiery, meat-eating
cardiac sloths
or helmet-less
paraplegic motorcyclists.

Maybe it's denial,
but coin flips and
rolling dice make
more sense to me.

March 13, 2009[3]

---

[3] Previously published in the 2011 edition of *Blood and Thunder: Musings on the Art of Medicine.*

I might have added this poem to my book even if I didn't think it belonged, just because it is one of the ones I like the best.

We are quite pleased that our oldest granddaughter, Kaitlyn, is playing on the University of Idaho women's golf team, less than 100 miles from our house in Moscow, Idaho. At 5'6" and 115 pounds, this beautiful, wiry athlete hits the ball much farther (and straighter) than most of the guys I know. She has had a wealth of tournament experience already, due to the vastly increased opportunities for girls and the dedication of her parents in providing the funds and time commitment for her activities and those of her sister, McKenzie (who made a hole-in-one just as I was giving this book a final proof).

Like most golfers, Kaitlyn still has work left to do on the mental aspects of her game. I keep my mouth shut in terms of golfing advice or coaching, except for one comment I made. I told her that in golf, the only shot you should think about is the one you are hitting at the moment. Let go of previous shots, guard against "shouldas" and "wouldas," and don't look forward to what you need to shoot on the remaining holes in order to score a certain score or beat another player. Stay in the present. This is the perfect place for using CBT methods to counter interfering, negative self-talk.

Even though I continue to work on not looking backward and second-guessing my actions (see "Assigning Blame" poem), I still get stuck with wondering about, and even castigating myself for, neglecting to go in for a rectal exam a year earlier when the cardiologist's office told me that my PSA had risen. (Remember that I had my PSA measured at the same time as my cholesterol level.) I'll keep working on this self-blame. Remember, I have spent my professional life teaching people to recognize and counter this sort of dysfunctional thinking. So don't feel bad if you find yourself with similar thoughts.

To Test or Not To Test?

A great deal of controversy has arisen recently about how soon, how often, and how routinely one should check PSA levels. In 2009, the American Urological Association (AUA) presented new guidelines for prostate cancer screening. Contrary to prior recommendations for screening to begin at age 50, with earlier screening for high-risk groups such as African Americans and men with a family history of prostate cancer, the AUA now suggests that men, who are first well informed and are at least 40 years of age and who have a life expectancy of at least 10 years, should be offered the PSA test to establish a baseline level. They suggest that rather than then having annual tests after 50, testing should be individualized. (Paddock 2009)

The AUA's rationale was that this baseline testing will lead to more curable cancers being found at an earlier stage. Otis Brawley, M.D., the Chief Medical Officer of the American Cancer Society, immediately disagreed, predicting that the implementation of baseline PSA testing will lead to unnecessary treatment. He said that the American Cancer Society did not recommend routine screening for all men. Instead, he advocated guidelines that ask doctors and patients to assess the potential benefits and risks of screening before deciding on a course of action (see Boyles 2009).

Watchful Waiting

Concerns over excess anxiety and unnecessary biopsies continue to provoke questions about prostate cancer screenings and bring renewed emphasis to "watchful waiting." Watchful waiting is a strategy of taking no action based on particular test results, while continuing to re-test on a regular basis. For example, one of my friends had an elevated PSA in his late 60s and chose watchful waiting. He had no therapy for several years and had his PSA levels checked regularly. When his PSA levels rose significantly, he underwent brachytherapy (placement of radioactive pellets in the prostate) and has been cancer-free for over a decade. If his PSA levels had remained the same, he would have likely been one of those who fit into the common category of, "Yes, you have prostate cancer, but you will most likely die of something else before it kills you."

Watchful waiting is also sometimes used with elevated or rising PSA levels before proceeding to a biopsy. Additionally, it is an option after a biopsy has detected cancer of the prostate. Depending on the estimated severity of the cancer, repeated assessments are done before proceeding to prostatectomy, some form of radiation therapy, hormone therapy, or some other treatment. Since prostate cancers vary widely in terms of aggressiveness, doctors use information such as measures of the degree of disorganization of the cells (i.e., the Gleason score) and PSA values in making treatment decisions. Of course, Gleason scores can only be known via biopsy.

Watchful waiting has the advantage of avoiding the cost and discomfort of unnecessary invasive procedures such as biopsies. It provides the same benefits for cases in which a given individual may remain symptom-free without any surgery or radiation. Of course, the tradeoff is that watchful waiting carries the risk of missing the window of opportunity for curing some cancers that might progress. It also keeps patients in the disquieting situation in which they have the unknown threat of cancer hanging over their heads.

I have a nephew whose father had prostate cancer. The nephew insisted that his physician screen him with PSA and rectal exam in his 40s, even though the physician told him it was unnecessary. His elevated PSA led to a positive biopsy and a prostatectomy. I also have a high school friend whose physician was reluctant to do a biopsy after his PSA rose. My friend insisted that the test be done. When the biopsy was positive, he was unwilling to put up with the uncertainty of watchful waiting and had a prostatectomy in his late 50s. Both men were pleased that they were assertive about what they wanted. Everyone has to make his own decisions, but the days of unquestioning acquiescence to medical authority have been transitioning to an era of collaborative decision-making between doctor and patient.

Conditions other than prostate cancer have been approached with watchful waiting for decades. For example, Dad was diagnosed with an abdominal aortic aneurism (AAA) when he was in his early 60s. AAA is an enlargement of the massive artery that carries oxygen-rich blood from the heart to the lower parts of the body. The problem with aneurisms anywhere in the body is that they weaken the vessel and can burst, resulting in strokes if they are in the brain, and quite frequently in death when they involve the aorta. Dad's cardiologist suggested watchful waiting, and for nearly two decades he performed an annual echocardiogram tracking the size of the aneurism. Though reportedly much improved in recent years, the surgery to repair an AAA is brutal.

I'm glad Dad did not have the surgery. I think it is likely that he would not have bounced back from it, and his quality of life would have been reduced. I say this despite the fact that a rupture of his AAA was almost certainly the cause of his death. The AAA had continued to grow to the point that, if he had been 53 or even 63 rather than 83, the doctors would have suggested surgery. But he lived to be 83 years old. He had Parkinson's disease, congestive heart failure, a cardiac pacemaker, and coronary artery disease that required something like nine angioplasties and several stents.

My sister had accompanied Dad on the plane from California to celebrate Thanksgiving with us in 2002. He took a fall the first day at our house and spent half the night in the emergency room being evaluated. The rest of the night, I slept near him and sat up with him while he complained of back pain. The next morning, I went to work for a half-day, anticipating four and a half days off with him over Thanksgiving. Our children and grandchildren were due in from Seattle and Portland the next day. In the middle of the session with my second psychotherapy client, I was interrupted by a call on our inside phone line. It was Karen telling me she thought Dad was dead, and that the ambulance was on its way. I nearly threw the poor lady with whom I was working out the door, yelled at my partner, Ginger, through her closed office door, and ran to my truck. I drove way too fast the four miles home, jumped out of the truck next to the fire truck, and stumbled into the house.

Karen said she had helped Dad back from the bathroom. After she guided him back into the recliner we had bought for his visit, he said, "Oh, oh, my back," and quickly became totally unresponsive. So the burst vessel had killed him after watchful waiting. While we were all profoundly sad that he'd died and especially that he had missed seeing the kids by just one day, he had a pretty good death. I'm sure the pain was extremely intense, but it only lasted a few seconds, and he died with people around him who loved him. I think watchful waiting was a good strategy for this condition for him. Also, he never did have surgery or radiation for prostate cancer. As with the aneurism, it is questionable as to whether Dad would have been able to tolerate a prostatectomy or radiation therapy without dramatically reducing his quality of life. The cancer was held at bay for over a decade with hormone therapy, and, despite the side effects, I think this less aggressive treatment was a good decision for him.

This week, the first of May 2011, two prostate cancer articles appeared in our local paper, *The Spokesman Review*. The first described new software program titled "VividLook" that, when used with magnetic resonance imaging techniques, promises to reduce the need for biopsies in some men, and make the biopsies that are done more useful.

The second article reported a long-term outcome study from Sweden. In a sample of 70 men, surgery rather than watchful waiting lowered the risk of dying of prostate cancer within 15 years by 38 percent, but the effect was significant only for men younger than 65. The title of the article was "Surgery for Early Prostate Cancer Helps Men under 65, Study Shows," which I found somewhat misleading. Well, maybe not misleading and certainly not deliberately so, but less relevant to men in the United States than the title might imply.

You see, in Europe, watchful waiting is much more frequently followed than it is in the United States. Prostate cancer in most of the men in this study was diagnosed only after clear symptoms, such as blood in the urine or semen; back, hip, or thigh pain; or difficulty with erections had occurred. In the United States, prostate cancer is overwhelmingly diagnosed after a PSA test has prompted a biopsy. Such a cancer in the United States is thus detected much earlier than it would be if one waited until overt symptoms appeared. Because the diagnosis that prompts treatment in the two countries is arrived at by such dramatically different methods, it is hard to judge what the Swedish data tell us about the wisdom of early treatment of prostate cancer in the United States.

The article noted that there were two long-term studies comparing watchful waiting as opposed to surgery in progress in the United States, using men whose prostate cancers had been first suspected because of elevated PSA readings. Such studies should provide results that are more easily interpreted, because the diagnostic methods will be comparable.

Finally, an article on the website cancernetwork.com on 8/12/11 reported development of a new prostate cancer diagnostic test refinement that involves measuring some substances in urine which relate to genes that function as an "on" switch for cancer of the prostate. They hope this test, the details of which were beyond my level of knowledge and need not be elaborated here, can be combined with other factors (I assume PSA level and PSA velocity as examples) to improve the accuracy of prediction of finding cancer in biopsies. Obviously, non-invasive tests that only require peeing in a cup are attractive if they increase predictability. I'm certain we will see a continuing search for the most efficient, least invasive diagnostic tests.

Given all of these differences of opinion and the appearance of evermore precise diagnostic methods, the wisest course seems to me to consult with your family doctor. If he tells you it is important to check your PSA given your age, family history, and general health, take his advice seriously, but do not blindly accept this recommendation. Use it as a starting point to study, ask questions, and become actively involved in this decision.

Abundance of Options: A Double-Edged Sword

The watchful waiting approach taken with Dad fits well with that advocated in a provocative book with a rather polemic title. Written by a cultural anthropologist who has been dealing with prostate cancer for 20 years in conjunction with his medical oncologist, *Invasion of the Prostate Snatchers* (Blum and Scholz 2009) comes down quite hard on the side of fewer rather than more biopsies, and less rather than more treatment of prostate cancer, especially for low and even moderate risk cases.

Blum and Scholz strongly advocate greatly increased reliance on time-limited, intermittent hormonal therapy. Also called intermittent androgen-suppression therapy, this approach involves taking hormones that block male hormones when the PSA has risen, but before any cancer symptoms develop. The treatment is interrupted after the PSA drops, and is reinstated when the PSA rises again. One huge problem with this approach is that there is a population of prostate cancer cells that is not affected by hormone therapy, and these are the same cells that are most likely to kill you. Walsh and Worthington (2007) noted that there is no empirical evidence that this approach increases progression-free survival, yet the patient has to endure the serious medical and quality-of-life impairments from the hormones. They also note that as of 2007, the American Society of Clinical Oncology considered intermittent androgen-suppression therapy to be experimental.

I'm happy with the title I chose for my book, but having "Invasion of the Prostate Snatchers" emblazoned on the cover and in the advertising copy for a book must be worth a few thousand sales, even if the book isn't much good. I didn't see this book until three years after my surgery, so I'm not certain that it would have influenced my decision to have surgery. It might have if my cancer was of a lower grade (lower Gleason score, slower increase in PSA, etc.), especially if I had been a decade older at the time, but not with my more aggressive cancer and younger age.

Today, there is a huge amount of information that is readily available concerning various diseases and their treatments, and this includes prostate cancer. Your local bookstore and library contain entire shelves devoted to these topics. The Internet has multiplied the number of sources anyone can access for free, just by entering the words prostate cancer into a search engine. You can easily find sites such as those sponsored by the American Urological Association, American Cancer Society, American Society of Clinical Oncology, Prostate Cancer Foundation, and National Cancer Institute.

The Edges of the Sword—A frustrating thing about prostate cancer is that there are a variety of treatment options. It can be overwhelming to try to investigate the different therapies and feel that you have made the right decision.

An encouraging thing about prostate cancer is that there are a variety of treatment options. As a first-line treatment, a man now can pick between several surgical and radiation therapies that all have excellent outcomes. And again, he often has watchful waiting as a reasonable option, under some circumstances.

We usually think that having many options from which to choose is a good thing. In fact, one way to measure the concept of freedom is in terms of the number of choices a person has—the more choices, the more freedom. And we all want freedom, right?

A fascinating book by Barry Schwartz, *The Paradox of Choice* (2004), is instructive in this regard. Schwartz is one of a number of authors who do a great service to the general reading public. Hardly any of us will dig through the latest scientific literature in medicine, psychology, sociology, social psychology, biology, and neurology to gather the sorts of information that these authors organize and present in an accurate but understandable and entertaining manner.

Along with Schwartz's book, I heartily recommend *Blink* (2007) and *The Tipping Point* (2000) by Malcolm Gladwell, *Learned Optimism* (1991) and *Authentic Happiness* (2002) by Martin E. P. Seligman, *How We Decide* by Jonah Lehrer (2009), and *Stumbling on Happiness* by Daniel Gilbert (2005).

Schwartz details the ways in which modern life has increased the number of options we face in every area and suggests that this is not necessarily a positive development. He contends that the vast amount of choice in modern life is, in fact, a major source of stress. The overabundance of choice may even detract from how satisfied we are with whatever choice we end up making. For example, Schwartz reports research in which students were shown either six or thirty gourmet chocolates. They then tasted one from the group. Finally, they were given a choice between payment for participating in the study or a small box of chocolates. Those who had been shown thirty chocolates rated the chocolate they tasted lower and more often picked the money rather than the box of chocolates, when compared to those shown only six chocolates. Increasing the number of choices of prostate cancer treatments may not lead to men being more satisfied with their choices.

Maybe even more importantly, what does research in this area say about factors influencing the quality of the choices that we make? As I have indicated, in my research for this book I have spent a large amount of time reading and thinking about decision-making and have found Lehrer's book cited above to be particularly intriguing. I have a hard time deciding how much detail to include here. I'll make do with a sampling, though it is tempting to list example after example from his book, and that is a tribute to his writing.

Lehrer makes a strong case for paying attention to which part of our brain we use for different sorts of decisions. He challenges the conventional view that the optimal approach to decision-making is to analyze your choices by doing a cost-benefit analysis. Instead, he cautions us to be aware of the sort of decision we are making, and to be sure to use the part of the brain that is best suited to that sort of decision-making. A great deal of research has compared performance in choosing when areas such as the orbitofrontal cortex and ventral striatum of the brain predominate, with the performance which occurs when brain structures that operate without the conscious awareness associated with these structures are primary.

Let's look at one of Lehrer's examples. Suppose you are tasked with choosing the best one out of four used cars, after being given four pieces of information about each car. If, after a few minutes of rational thought, you are asked to choose, you will do fairly well, picking the best choice about half the time. Repeat the task, but this time you are immediately distracted from the choice, so that your "unconscious/emotional" brain has to choose. In this situation, you will perform much more poorly.

Now let's increase the difficulty of the task. Rather than being given only four factors, you are told a dozen things about each vehicle. You are then asked to think about it for a short time, while allowing the rational brain to do its thing. In this case, you will do worse than you would merely by random guessing. But if you are distracted so that only the emotional brain is in play, you will do quite well, picking the best car about 60 percent of the time.

I find it fascinating that Lehrer also describes experiments illustrating that the emotional brain makes these decisions long before we have any conscious awareness. By coincidence, an article appeared in this morning's (June 21, 2011) edition of *The Spokesman Review* entitled "Study Links Teen Brain To Success Of Pop Songs." In 2006, neuroeconomist (didn't know there was such a thing, huh?) Gregory Berns measured the brain activity of a group of teenagers while they listened to some new music from somewhat obscure artists. Since it was already known that the activity in the orbitofrontal cortex and ventral striatum areas of our brain can predict what we will choose, the question asked was, "Would the brain activity of this group predict which songs the general population of teens would actually buy?" The brain scans predicted with 90 percent accuracy which songs would flop and which would succeed. Remarkably, the teens' conscious ratings of the songs were completely unrelated to the probability that the songs would succeed. Again, the value of listening to the emotional brain was confirmed.

It's as though when inundated with too much information, the rational brain becomes so overwhelmed by extraneous information that it may not be the most important mechanism with regard to making the best choice. Lehrer notes that it is as if we are, ". . . trying to run a new computer program on an old machine." (p.158)

So it seems that with simpler problems, it is wise to spend a fair amount of time thinking things over, but with more complex problems, it is wise to trust the immediate reaction of the emotional brain.

Long after I had made my decision to have surgery, in fact, over a year after I had the surgery, I began reviewing research in this area of decision-making with special attention to making choices about prostate cancer treatment. As I have read about the importance of the emotional brain, I have wondered if my extensive study of prostate cancer and its treatment may not have been such a good idea after all. Maybe I would have been better off "just going with how I felt" at the time.

It is important to note that in cases where the emotional brain is superior, the "supercomputer" that is the emotional brain has been prepared by past experience. Lehrer notes that novel problems (i.e., ones with which a person has not had much experience) benefit from the use of reason. For example, novice golfers do better if they spend time studying various factors about the green before they putt, but after repeated practice, golfers do better without a great deal of conscious input. They are better off listening to their unconscious emotional brain.

As I have been thinking about my decision-making, I have reminded myself that most of us have not had a great deal of experience in wading through medical information in order to make treatment decisions. Thus, maybe it is reasonable to see choices in this area as presenting novel problems. And since there really were only two choices for me—surgery and external-beam radiation therapy—because brachytherapy and watchful waiting were clearly eliminated as reasonable choices by the doctors, maybe the decision can be seen as a "simple" problem in that regard, though with a fair amount of background noise created by the amount I read about the disease.

I am still unclear as to whether the emotional or rational brain is the best choice for decisions such as prostate cancer treatment. However, one instance in which I do agree with Lehrer is in terms of the importance of "thinking about your thinking." An analysis of your own decision-making can be an important guard against placing too much weight on one method versus another in an area in which that might not be optimal.

My current thinking is that I probably did a good job of thinking about my thinking. I was talking to myself and to others, in particular Karen and Bill, about what I had learned, what I thought about, what I had read, and how I was feeling about it. Then, after all of the conscious research, it's as though I let my emotional brain make the decision. How is that? Well, after rummaging all the information around in my skull for weeks, one night I went to sleep, and when I woke up, I knew that I wanted to have the surgery done in Spokane by Rob Golden. In the end, I think I listened to the supercomputer of the emotional brain, which was doing its thing while I slept.

I'm also fairly certain not only that it would have been very difficult for me to avoid gathering information about my disease, but also that I would not have been satisfied that I had been responsible if I had not done so. That's just the way I am.

Of course, for many illnesses there aren't a number of options that are nearly the same in terms of outcome, so there isn't much of a decision to be made. For many people, the decision boils down to whether to do what the doctor suggests, or do nothing. The world has changed dramatically in the last few decades, however. In *The Paradox of Choice,* Schwartz summarizes the change in healthcare as follows: "The tenor of medical practice has shifted from one in which the all-knowing, paternalistic doctor tells the patient what must be done—or just does it—to one in which the doctor arrays the possibilities before the patient . . . and the patient makes a choice." (2004, p. 3)

Yes, we all want freedom, and we think that more choices will make us happier. In this regard, I refer you also to *Stumbling on Happiness*, in which Gilbert makes clear that we often have little clue as to how we will react to events and cannot predict with much accuracy what will make us happy. Finally, Lehrer reports on the writing of Atul Gawande, a physician who has taken a great interest in this area. Gawande reported that a great many patients prefer to have others make their treatment decisions, rather than having the responsibility for doing so themselves. Sixty-five percent of people surveyed said that they would want to choose their own treatment if they contracted cancer. However, among people who actually get cancer, only 12 percent choose to pick their own treatment.

Of course, if having many possible treatments for prostate cancer does raise the risk that a person will be dissatisfied with whatever he chooses, it is critical that each of us pays attention to how we talk to ourselves after our decisions, so that we do not heap unnecessary blame or regret on ourselves or others—regardless of what we choose, and whatever the outcome of that choice.

The Bottom Line

In the end, as you will see while you continue to investigate prostate cancer, there are three Big Questions about treatment:

(1) Is this disease going to shorten my life? Will it kill me?

(2) If I have treatment, will I be able to control my urination afterward?

(3) If I have treatment, will I still be able to get erections afterward?

Let me address the first question here. Of course, each of us is concerned about how long we will continue to process oxygen, and how soon we might develop advanced disease if we are not "cured." What about long-term results from surgery or external-beam radiation therapy? Though Walsh has spent his life perfecting the anatomical (nerve-sparing) prostatectomy procedure, he states that national consensus panels currently consider both surgery and radiation techniques to be effective methods, which have somewhat different patterns of side effects.

Walsh has some reassuring words about the long-term benefits of surgery. First of all, he notes that if a man is in good health and is expected to live at least another 10 years, the side effects of radical prostatectomy are low enough that it makes sense to attempt a cure by doing the surgery. In the case of older men with a shorter expected lifetime remaining, the side effects from surgery are likely to be more severe. In such cases, he suggests that radiation is probably a better choice (2007, p. 201). Later, he notes that even for men whose cancer did metastasize after surgery, the average time for this to occur from when the man's PSA first increased after surgery was eight years, and 82 percent of men who had a post-surgical PSA rise did not have metastatic cancer by the time 15 years had passed since their surgery. Even then, men lived an average of five more years.

Surgery is an excellent treatment for prostate cancer, but when all is said and done, there is no one best choice in terms of chances for a cure for all individuals.

Improvements in a variety of prostate cancer treatment methods have allowed for dramatic changes in side effects, such as incontinence and erectile dysfunction, as discussed more fully in the FUTURE chapter. Note that throughout this book, I use the term "erectile dysfunction" rather than "impotence." The former is a descriptive term. The latter has too much extra baggage.

For example, *Webster's Encyclopedic Unabridged Dictionary* defines impotence as "lacking power or ability," "without force or effectiveness," "lacking bodily strength or physically helpless." It is a judgmental, pejorative word. The use of this term to describe one particular aspect of a man's functioning buys into the notion of measuring a man's worth, value or manliness in terms of whether or not blood pools in the spongy tissues of his penis. Surely one's masculinity, as well as one's worth is more than that. The most cowardly, the most selfish, the cruelest son-of-a-bitch may be able to achieve and maintain an erection the likes of which would make Trigger proud or give new meaning to the Lone Ranger's trademark cry of, "Hi-ho, Silver!"—yet we might not see him as much of a man in any important sense of the word.

Radiation and Other Consultations
When we first consulted with Dr. Golden, he described the various options for treatment and finished with the following table showing outcomes of surgery versus those of radiation therapy over time. The percentages refer to the probability of disease-free survival.

Time since	5 yrs	10 yrs	15 yrs
Surgery	95%	90%	85%
Radiation	90%	80%	30%

This table showed roughly comparable outcomes at five- and ten-year follow-ups, but a superiority of surgery over radiation at 15 years. That impressed me at the time, though further reading has suggested that the most likely conclusion is that there may be no substantial advantage of one over the other, even in the long run. This will probably become even clearer as more time passes with external-beam radiation therapy done with the aid of advanced imaging technology, which is making it much more effective. Because PSA levels drop very soon after prostatectomy, as opposed to a gradual decline over much longer periods with external-beam radiation therapy, direct comparisons of disease-free survival rates between the methods is difficult. There is now a great deal of evidence that both of these methods provide excellent results. I will return to this important issue in the chapter titled BIOCHEMICAL FAILURE—SALVAGE RADIATION.

Cutters wanna cut and zappers wanna zap. That's a cutesy way of saying that if you ask a urologist who is also a surgeon which treatment is best for prostate cancer, you'll most likely hear "prostatectomy," and if you ask a radiation oncologist, you'll most likely hear "radiation therapy." There also is the old caution of not asking your barber whether or not you need a haircut.

I think I was fortunate to be dealing with Dr. Golden. At the end of our first meeting, he gave us the names of two radiation oncologists and said that along with our reading, we should arrange a consultation with one of them before deciding on the path to follow. As I think back, getting another opinion didn't seem like a mere suggestion. He presented it as the next logical step that we would take to become informed before making a decision.

I have talked to a number of men and read of numerous cases where newly-diagnosed, panicky patients received rather abrupt, dismissive treatment by urologists who merely told them what they needed to do, with this declaration sometimes accompanied by dire predictions of death from prostate cancer within some specific time period if they did not have that specific treatment. The sort of spirit of collaboration engendered by Dr. Golden makes more sense in the modern age. It also fits with the advice of Patrick Walsh, who says to get a second opinion before entering into treatment of prostate cancer.

Our next consultation a week after meeting with Dr. Golden was with Dr. Christopher Lee, one of the radiation oncologists Dr. Golden recommended. It's notable that, as did Dr. Golden, Dr. Lee asked me to bring Karen to our meeting. That may just be standard practice, but I thought it showed sensitivity and compassion.

Dr. Lee was a pleasant young man who chatted with us as he took a history. When it came time for the rectal exam, he asked if I wanted to have Karen wait outside. Never particularly modest and seeing it as routine, I said she might as well stay. He asked us about our sexual life, and I remember remarking that we continued to make love without any particular difficulty, though I noted that the last time we both cried part of the time while doing so, because of my diagnosis. In answering our questions about outcomes, he proudly called up on his computer some of the research studies he had co-authored, including one which compared radiation and surgery for prostate cancer, and which was the largest to date in terms of number of subjects involved. His work showed no difference in outcomes between the two treatments.

As he was asking us about where I had gone to school and where we had lived, we learned that he, too, had studied at Utah State University before finishing his undergraduate degree at Brigham Young University. His grandfather had been teaching in the chemistry department at USU while I was there. We traded stories of our time in Logan. Small world.

We thought it was significant that he spent nearly two hours with us. He did take a couple of brief phone calls, which seemed reasonable. During one of his phone breaks, Karen broke the tension with some of the sort of inside humor that people in long-time relationships are wont to develop: "This probably isn't a good time to tell him about your letter demanding to be excommunicated from the Mormon Church." Fortunately, we were able to stop laughing before he returned. I, of course, chose not to share that story or my reasons for formally leaving that institution, with which I had not been involved since I was 12 years old.

As usual, I came in with a long list of specific questions about Dr. Lee, his training and experience, and various radiation treatment alternatives. Dr. Lee provided easily understandable descriptions of external-beam radiation therapy and brachytherapy ("seeds"). He noted that my cancer was a bit too advanced for brachytherapy. He told us about the improvements in external-beam radiation therapy, especially as related to the use of improved imaging devices for more accurate targeting. These developments allow more of the radiation to hit the areas it needs to destroy, while decreasing the spread of damage to healthy tissue.

Dr. Lee described a regimen of 41 treatments over eight weeks. First, though, the shape of the prostate in three dimensions would be mapped using a CT scan. Based on this information, an individualized radiation treatment plan, called conformal radiation, would be devised by Dr. Lee and a team, which included a person with a Ph.D. in physics. A plastic cast of my body would be made that would hold me in the same position for each treatment. The body cast and a repeat CT scan prior to each treatment are designed to improve the targeting of the prostate. I had never thought about it, but apparently the organs inside each of us do shift a bit from one moment to the next. He also said that because of the combination of my PSA and Gleason scores, I would need a course of hormone treatments for a period of time before the radiation began.

Radiation treatments lead to side effects such as fatigue, painful skin reactions (sleeping on lamb's wool during the two months of therapy was recommended by several people), and various bladder and bowel symptoms that ranged from mild to severe. Everything I have read suggests that the side effects fade as time passes after the final treatment, with bowel and bladder problems the most likely to persist. Long-term difficulties with erectile dysfunction and incontinence appear to be comparable to those caused by radical prostatectomy.

One important difference is that with radical prostatectomy, erectile function improves for up to a year or more after surgery, as the mechanical trauma to important nerves and blood vessels that support erections heals over time. Within a few weeks after radiation therapy is completed, erectile function returns, but at that time it is as good as it's going to be. Over time, damage to the nerves and blood vessels from the radiation treatment progresses, often leading to gradually decreasing function. Also, with the surgery, the information about PSA level is available after only a few weeks; whereas with radiation, PSA levels drop gradually over a much longer period, leading to an extended period of uncertainty.

Obviously, none of this information about these options was pleasant. Neither was the thought of surgery. However, the procedure that seemed to gross me out the most was a particular type of brachytherapy. Remember that regular brachytherapy involves the implantation of rice-sized radioactive seeds in a cancerous prostate and is noted to be an effective treatment in cases where it is deemed appropriate. It is less invasive, has a quicker recovery time than surgery, and irradiates far less healthy tissue than external-beam radiation therapy. A series of small tubes is inserted up through your perineum and into the prostate, precise placement guided by imaging techniques. You are anesthetized, and then the seeds are inserted. You wake up and go home in a day or so. Pretty nifty—no scars, quick recovery. Even though I was not a candidate for brachytherapy of any kind, Dr. Lee also detailed a new alternative brachytherapy technique. Maybe he just wanted us to know all possible options.

Rather than going home after the seeds are implanted as in regular brachytherapy, this new technique involved a four-day hospital stay. Why four days, you ask? They are just sticking the seeds in there, right? Well, in this case, they put you under, then insert a number of cannulas through your perineum (think tiny soda straws just to the front of your anus) into which they insert the radioactive pellets. Only this time, when you come out of the anesthetic, you are lying there with the cannulas still sticking out of your perineum. You lie there like that for the four days, after which the cannulas are removed and you go home.

But, wait, wait, wait—here's the best part. Then you return to the hospital a couple of weeks later, and they repeat the process. No incision or anastamosis to heal, as with a radical retropubic prostatectomy, and much quicker than a 41-day course of external-beam radiation treatments, but either seemed preferable to me at the time. Somehow, I was reminded of what we used to say as kids to make our buddies squirm, "Imagine that you are sliding down a banister and it turns into a razor blade." Whether due to that image or not, that part of my anatomy seems rather vulnerable to me (maybe because **IT IS**).

In any case, the prospect of regaining consciousness with a porcupine sprouting from the bottom of my crotch and having to lie there for a several days was too much for me. There aren't enough mind-altering drugs in the hospital pharmacy to get me through that one. After all, as I describe later, I had a difficult time warding off a panic attack when I was in the hospital for an angiogram. At that time, I was tethered to an IV, but that was much less restrictive than Mr. Porcupine would be.

Before I discuss a couple of other very promising forms of radiation therapy, I want to make note of something pretty basic that you might not have considered. I had never asked the question of exactly why radiation works as a cancer treatment. I mean, the doctors and their assistants are blasting away in there to kill the cancer cells. What about all the healthy cells? Aren't they wiped out at the same time? It is a fortunate fact that radiation is most harmful to cells that are growing rapidly. Guess which cells are growing the most rapidly? Yep. Cancer cells. Those little devils grow much faster than healthy cells. This wild, runaway growth is the source of the damage done to the body by cancer.

However, it is also a benefit, because the cancer cells are going to sustain much more damage than the nearby, slower-growing, healthy cells, even if both receive the same dose of radiation. Add this phenomenon to the progressively improving imaging techniques that allow for more specific targeting of cancer cells versus normal cells, and you end up with fewer and milder side effects than ever before.

Radiation treatment of prostate cancer has been revolutionized by the availability of increasingly accurate imaging techniques. The goal of all these radiation treatments is to deliver the maximum dose of radiation to the cancerous tissues while doing the least damage to surrounding healthy tissues. Early radiation therapy for prostate cancer looked good, until it was discovered that it resulted in active cancer remaining in a large percentage of men who thought they had been cured. To avoid damage to adjacent organs, such as the bladder and rectum, the size of the radiation dosage being administered was not sufficiently high to wipe out all the cancer. The higher the dosage, the greater the damage to the DNA of the cells.

Fortunately, the newer imaging methods allow more precise, three-dimensional views of the size, shape, and location of the prostate. First came three-dimensional, conformal radiation therapy (3-DCRT) with CT scanning, and then later, intensity-modulated radiation therapy (IMRT) with more sophisticated computer and imaging techniques that enabled the medical team to match their radiation beams more closely to the boundaries of each man's prostate.

With all of these methods, a plaster cradle or cast, such as the one Dr. Lee described, is molded for each person to hold his body in the same position during each session of radiation. However, even with this precaution, there is room for error in the delivery of the radiation beam, due to moment-to-moment movements of the prostate produced by breathing and changes in the contents of the bladder or gas in the rectum.

Cyberknife®—The quest for more accurate targeting of prostate cancer led to the development of the CyberKnife® Robotic Radiosurgery System, which one of my high school friends, Chuck, recently chose in place of a prostatectomy. The CyberKnife® uses a computer-controlled robotic arm to deliver radiation from a variety of directions to different parts of the prostate. Except for a minimally-invasive outpatient procedure reminiscent of a prostate biopsy, in which a few tiny gold seeds called fiducials or fiducial markers are placed in the prostate, this is a non-invasive procedure.

These fiducials are used along with real-time, moment-to-moment X-ray imaging to identify the exact position of the prostate each time the robotic arm is moved to a new position. If the prostate has shifted slightly, the path of the radiation beam is adjusted accordingly. Because knowledge of the position of the target allows the delivery of higher doses of photon radiation with less collateral damage, this therapy is completed in just one to five sessions.

As I write this section, it has been two months since my friend Chuck had five sessions, and he is doing quite well, though he continues to experience significant rectal symptoms. His doctor said they have a 100% cure rate at their facility so far, but acknowledged that they didn't expect that record to hold up over time.

Proton Therapy—Several years ago, another of my friends spent two months at Loma Linda Medical Center in California to undergo proton therapy, another non-invasive form of radiation cancer treatment that is unique, because it uses protons rather than photons to attack the malignant cells. Advocates of this approach point to the fact that, because of the nature of protons, when a proton beam is sent into the body, it delivers the vast majority of its energy at a specific location, with little radiation energy deposited either during its journey to the target or to tissues beyond the target.

Because photon radiation spends part of its energy as it passes through the body to the targeted cancer cells, the photon beam has to be much stronger than proton radiation in order to deliver enough radiation to kill the cancer cells. More radiation to more tissue leads to more collateral damage, and thus, proton therapy purportedly produces fewer side effects than photon-based therapy, though this latter claim is disputed by some. I did not hear about proton therapy until several months after my surgery. (Actually, there is a single paragraph in Walsh's book, but it must not have registered with me.)

As I read about proton therapy on a variety of websites, I was struck with how closely bonded many of the men who had received proton therapy had become. Much of this closeness may have been due to the fact that they usually live together at the treatment site for the duration of their treatment, since there are a limited number of sites around the country. They have considerable time together in this setting, including participation in regular support groups. I was somewhat put off by the near-evangelical use of testimonials on the websites, such as one touting the BOB, or "Brotherhood of the Balloon." Apparently, the proton therapy protocol requires the insertion of some sort of a balloon in the rectum every day for the treatment, as a way to reduce movement of the prostate during the radiation session.

One aspect of proton radiation therapy that causes concern is its enormous cost, which I have heard quoted as from $65,000 to $135,000, due to the $200 million in construction expense for a linear accelerator.

I wondered if I was being overly critical or cynical in my reaction to this therapy. Since there was some mention of its now being used as a salvage radiation treatment, I thought I should at least check it out, in case I might need further treatment. "Salvage" is a term used for radiation therapy that is provided after surgical removal of the prostate, when PSA levels suggest that not all cancer cells were removed by the surgery.

Dr. Lee provided me with a review article by Nyguen, Trofimov and Zietman (2008) that compared proton beam therapy with IMRT. Nyguen et al. call for a randomized trial of IMRT versus proton therapy. They concluded that evidence for the superiority of proton therapy over conformal radiation approaches was inadequate. They stated that proton therapy should not be seen as more than a treatment with "tremendous promise" until such a trial was completed.

The Clinical Practice Guidelines recently published by the National Comprehensive Cancer Network conclude in a similar fashion that, "[P]roton therapy is not recommended for routine use at this time, since clinical trials have not yet yielded data that demonstrates superiority or equivalence of proton beam compared to conventional external beam for treatment of prostate cancer." (www.nccn.org, 2010, p. M-5-7) Beyers (2011) calls for comparative effectiveness research involving randomized clinical trials and a more clear demonstration that this therapy is worth the cost.

As I was reviewing my manuscript before submitting to the publisher, I read in the January 31, 2012, edition of *The Spokesman Review* about another proton therapy study which reported that proton therapy for prostate cancer led to one-third more bowel problems, including bleeding and blockages, than did conventional radiation methods. I'm sure more research in this area is planned.

The advances of 3-DCRT and IMRT clearly showed improved results over techniques lacking advanced imaging technology. New methods such as proton therapy and CyberKnife® offer great hope for the future. A number of ongoing controlled trials should tell us more about their long-term effectiveness.

On the website of the CyberKnife Centers of San Diego (www.sdcyberknife.com), there is a chart listing the advantages and disadvantages of CyberKnife® as compared to radical prostatectomy, external-beam radiation therapy, and brachytherapy. In this table are two notable summary statements: (1) "The long term curative potential of CyberKnife® radiosurgey remains to be defined," and (2) "Radical prostatectomy is the only local treatment method proven to increase overall survival in early stage prostate cancer patients." The latter statement probably refers to the 10-year follow up of the Swedish study I described earlier in this chapter.

It seems as though some people prefer the notion of prostatectomy, because it physically removes the cancer. This attitude may have played a part in my decision. However, there is no doubt now that the various radiotherapies are also very effective.

After the consultations with Dr. Golden and Dr. Lee, and extensive research on my own, I had gathered a rather large amount of information about my options. I called a urologist at the University of Washington Medical Center who was described as an expert surgeon. In a brief phone call, he said he would set up a consultation and estimated that the chances of my retaining the ability to have erections to be at least 80 percent. When I mentioned Dr. Golden's name, he said something like, "He must not do very many surgeries, because I have never had any consults referred by him." While this comment may have been nothing more than another example of the urban western Washington view that our side of the state is Hicksville, it didn't take long for me to decide not to schedule a meeting with him.

I also scheduled a visit with Dr. Rinaldi, our family doctor, and talked over my thought process with him to see if he believed I was approaching the decision in a reasonable manner. He assured me that he thought I was.

During this period of information-gathering and evaluation, I was calmed somewhat by Dr. Golden's report of a very large study that had just been completed, which showed no long-term difference in outcome between cases in which men had surgery right after diagnosis and cases in which men waited a period of several months. I needed to make a decision, but I did not need to rush. Since that time, I have talked with a number of men who were trying to decide on a treatment plan. In each case, they had a sense of urgency similar to that which I initially experienced.

Regarding the choice of surgery, I had read about laparoscopic and robotic methods, but I did not explore them in depth. They did seem to offer the possibility of a slightly shorter hospital stay and recovery, and Dr. Golden had experience with the robot. However, I was impressed by his preference for being able to examine the lymph nodes directly with his fingers to assess the chances of metastases, which could not be done except with an open surgery.

It's probably just as well that I didn't spend much time on the wide variety of alternative therapies I have since read about. In the book *Invasion of the Prostate Snatchers,* Blum writes about such approaches he tried over the years, most of which have no evidence for their efficacy. I won't detail them here, since you can check out his book for the details. His co-author, Dr. Sholz, suggests that such strategies can still be useful, because of the power of the placebo effect to help people. While I am convinced as to the power of placebos in many areas of medicine and psychology, I am continuing to try to use only medical and ancillary approaches that have at least some science behind them.

Serendipity

I am repeatedly intrigued by the way in which seemingly chance events profoundly affect our lives. For instance, if I would not have driven down the hill on Rowan Avenue 51 years ago, I would not have waved at the gorgeous 15-year-old blonde who waved back and has been with me ever since. In my flailing around for information and opinions concerning prostate cancer treatment, I ran across a letter in my desk from Dad's cousin, Gary Maxwell. It dawned on me that Gary might be a helpful source regarding my decision.

A decade older than I am, Gary had been a kidney transplant surgeon in Salt Lake City, and later the head of a medical residency program at the University of North Carolina at Wilmington, with a specialty in trauma surgery. He and I had reconnected several years earlier when he was doing research for a Utah history book he was writing. Karen and I had even met him for lunch in the unlikely location of Beaver, Utah, when our travel paths coincided.

Gary emailed me right back saying that he had been out of medicine so long, he did not feel that he had up-to-date information that would be helpful. However, he reminded me that his son, Brian, who had stopped by our house with his dad for a visit the year before, was a third-year medical student at Stanford, the same university where two of my friends had gone for nerve-sparing surgery done by James Brooks, a protégé of Patrick Walsh. After Gary and Brian left our house, Karen and I had remarked that this humorous, socially-conscious young man was just the sort of person we wanted to see become a physician. As an added bonus, Brian's girlfriend (today his wife), Jen Liu, was a urology resident at Stanford.

I emailed Brian about my prostate cancer and the information that had been used in staging my disease. On Christmas Day, I received the first of several helpful emails containing Jen's opinions. I had been agonizing in particular as to whether to stay in Spokane or go to one of the big hospitals (coincidentally, Stanford was the one the most people were recommending). Jen noted that going to a teaching hospital almost guaranteed that at least part of the surgery would be performed by a resident, rather than by the surgeon. Brian discussed his own moral dilemma, seeing the serious need for training for himself, Jen, and all other medical students, yet being unwilling to have residents perform surgery on his own body. Jen summarized her view something like this: "I wouldn't recommend that my father or brother have the surgery done in a big teaching hospital. If you can find a local surgeon that you trust and can communicate with, who has done at least 500 of the surgeries and does at least 50 a year, choose that person." So now I had more information and opinions to chew on. I appreciated Jen's kindness and her frank opinion.

At Last, a Decision

Even if you have not had to make a decision about treatment for a life-threatening disease, you may have had an experience similar to mine regarding making a choice about something important, be it a vacation, one automobile or another, which woman to marry, or which career to pursue. Frequently, when trying to decide between one course of action and another, I have made lists of pros and cons for each choice, even given weights of importance to options. Invariably, there has not been one clear winner. That certainly was the case with prostate cancer treatment. I suppose if there were a single correct answer, I wouldn't be having so much difficulty making a choice. It would be clear.

I used to tell psychotherapy clients that when a choice between two options was so difficult that the pros and cons seemed to come out even, they could be pretty sure that they'd be okay with either choice. In those instances, it's not like you are choosing between a week-long ménage a trois in Paris with Julia Roberts and Penelope Cruz, or having a rusty ice pick jammed into your eyeball.

My being stuck illustrates another example of irrational automatic self-talk. In this instance, A, the Activating Event, was the situation of needing to choose a treatment. B probably was self-talk such as, *There is a best choice, one right answer here. I must not make a mistake by choosing something other than the perfect path to follow.* C, of course, was anxiety and the resulting inertia. In fact, I needed to counter these self-defeating ideas, to tell myself that there was no one right, perfect choice.

That's just not the way it is with prostate cancer today. I had more than one very reasonable option, each proven to be effective, though with somewhat different side effects. I really couldn't make a mistake. Being able to tolerate ambiguity in a situation like this, where there is no single correct answer, is crucial. I'm not sure that I did as good a job of countering my self-defeating automatic thoughts at the time as I have indicated here in hindsight, but I did make a decision.

In truth, with difficult decisions, it seems that I often gather a bunch of information, then end up "going with my gut" or "following my heart," and that's what I ended up doing regarding the choice of surgery versus radiation therapy.

As I said before, after I had done extensive research and let it rattle around in my mind for a while, I woke up one December morning with the clear decision to have the surgery done in Spokane by Dr. Golden. Maybe it was a case of going with my gut after lots of preparing with my brain.

Anatomical (Nerve-Sparing) Surgery

I had seen repeated descriptions of the improved techniques invented by Dr. Patrick Walsh. I was astounded to learn that before 1987, no one had identified the location of the nerves that control erections. Walsh tackled the problem while working with another urologist in Sweden that year. He said that some anatomy texts had suggested that, while they had not located the nerves in question, they must run through the prostate gland itself. Walsh thought this was unlikely, since he knew of no other gland in the body where the nerves ran through it in this way.

Working with stillborn males, he located the nerves running a few millimeters away from and along each side of the prostate. These nerves trigger relaxation in the veins in the penis to allow blood to engorge the columns of spongy tissue and create an erection. No wonder so many men in the past experienced erectile dysfunction following prostatectomies. The tiny nerves were undoubtedly being hacked out of there when the prostate was removed.

Walsh developed a method for excising the prostate while sparing the nerves. He repeatedly videotaped his surgeries to perfect his procedure. Thousands of men (and their partners) have him to thank for their continuing ability to have intercourse following a prostatectomy. I'm sure every one of those guys would agree that Walsh's has been an example of "a life well-lived."

Dr. Golden had done his first prostatectomy during his residency at the University of Oregon. Patrick Walsh was visiting the facility that summer, so Dr. Golden's first prostatectomy was an anatomical or nerve-sparing one, done with the surgeon who invented the procedure.

More Decisions and Preparation

After deciding to follow the path of surgery for my cancer, the next logical step was to choose a hospital. As I was talking with Dr. Golden, he said something about doing the majority of his prostatectomies at Valley Hospital and Medical Center, located just a few miles from my house. Without thinking, I said something like, "Okay, let's just do it there." He had a time open in a late January, so we scheduled the procedure. For whatever reason, I was soon ambivalent about that choice. Then while I was running with my friend, Bill, he said that he would choose the facility that did the largest number of this type of surgery. His comment fit in with my thoughts, and with the recommendations that I had read.

My initial internal reaction was, *I don't want to inconvenience Dr. Golden and his office.* I soon countered that thinking with something more reasonable and called him back. He did not hesitate for a second. "It's completely up to you, your choice. I don't like to do surgeries on Fridays, as I may not be on call and available on the weekend to follow up, but I have January 29th open." Even though that was my granddaughter Kaitlyn's 15th birthday, I committed to that date. I immediately felt relieved. This choice and Dr. Golden's ready accommodation of my wishes is another example of a way I was able to feel like I had some control over what was happening to me.

Sometime in December, when Bill and I were on another run, he said something on the order of, "You should use this time before your surgery to get in the best shape possible, adding various calisthenics to your running." Now, I have always been someone who would prefer going for a long run to spending even a half hour lifting weights or doing other strength-building exercises. However, this seemed like a no-lose proposition.

I began doing sit-ups and push-ups and a few other exercises every day, using my running diary to chart my progress. Who knows, maybe this regimen helped my recovery, allowing me to maneuver more efficiently as I healed. Since they cut through abdominal muscles to get to the prostate, strengthening that area might have helped in recovery. I also made it a point every day to do the Kegel exercises to strengthen muscles used in controlling the flow of urine. I'll discuss these exercises further in the SURGERY chapter. As I thought about Bill's suggestion, I also realized that whether or not it had any benefit, the exercise regimen was providing me with a degree of control in yet another area of my life.

So, one of my main messages to you is to do as much research as fits best with you and your desires. Take whatever steps you can to control important aspects of your life, including your physical condition. Then, when you are as informed as is comfortable for you, make the decision that seems best for you, and don't for a second look back. Second guesses will not help. In the RECOVERY chapter, I will discuss at length our inevitable limits on being able to control important things about our health. Acceptance is the companion of Control. Some combination of the two is required for optimum adjustment.

We celebrated Kaitlyn's birthday in Portland a week early. When we were ready to leave for home, with just two days before the surgery, the weather turned sour. The Columbia River Gorge was closed, with vehicles strewn across the snow-filled road and no opening in sight. Great, it appeared that we couldn't get back to Spokane in time for the surgery on Tuesday. We decided to drive up I-5 to Seattle, then across I-90 over Snoqualmie Pass through the Cascade Mountains to Spokane. Usually, it would be Snoqualmie that would be the problem. This detour would add several hours to the trip, but we could stop and have lunch with our son Steven and his wife, Sue, outside of Seattle. We saved them some postage, too, because they had an elaborate post-surgical care package for me, including books, puzzles, snacks, and a tray that could hold our laptop computer. Not a bad idea to visit both of the kids and their families right before major surgery, anyway. Their concern and support was much appreciated, as were the telephone calls from my sister Lynne and brother Kerry.

3

SURGERY

When dealing with a decision such as which way to treat a life-threatening disease, it is very easy to become so self-absorbed that you lose touch with how this process is affecting the important people in your life. And it is affecting them, even if you are oblivious to that fact. In the middle of my worry about myself, it dawned on me that I would be in the operating room for several hours while Karen sat alone. I called her running buddy, Paula Vandenburg, an obstetrics nurse, and asked her if she could keep Karen company during the procedure.

Despite some scheduling conflicts, Paula showed up on the morning of my surgery. I remember seeing her with Karen when I got back in a fog from the post-op recovery room. I know Karen was grateful for her support. I was reminded once more that it is a good thing to get out of yourself sometimes.

At 7 a.m., right before we went into the pre-op room where they check your vital signs, ask you repeatedly why you are there, have you sign some more papers, and start an IV, a smiling face of Scots-Irish heritage peeked around the corner. Jack McBride had left his hometown of Colfax, 60 miles south of Spokane, before 5:30 in the morning to sit with Karen while I was in surgery. I should have known. Pals since age 10, he and I have shared over half a century of life's travels. A retired school teacher and coach, Jack is the friendliest, most kind person you will meet. He is also a person who lives his Christian faith as fully as anyone I have known, yet does so without trying to ram Jesus down your throat.

A nurse, then a nurse anesthetist, and finally the anesthesiologist each took a whack at getting an IV into my arm. During this process, someone asks who Jack is. The answer: "My brother from Colfax."

"Oh, Okay.

"Out of the corner of my eye, I see Karen and Jack trying to suppress giggles. You see, I am tall and thin enough that friends said I should insist on the "skinny guy discount" from Dr. Golden, since it will be so easy for him to get to where he needs to go in my abdomen—and Jack is a fireplug. Not exactly Arnold Schwarzenegger and Danny Devito in the movie *Twins*, but an unlikely brother pair.

It just goes to show you, though. Act like you know what you are doing, and you can get along just fine. I did that often when teaching classes to very sharp undergraduate and graduate students in psychology. If I began to feel intimidated when I thought of how little I actually knew about a lot of things, it helped greatly to remind myself that about the subject of that day's class, I probably knew a hell of a lot more than the best of them. If you throw in a willingness to say, "I don't know," when you don't have a freaking clue, you can sail along and teach students a great deal, even when you have less than great expertise.

The trio of experts in phlebotomy did not succeed in establishing an open conduit into any veins in my arm. The last one to try decided to use a vein in my neck, an option that did not turn out well for me due to agonizing spasms in my neck for several days after surgery.

I knew they'd be shaving my lower abdomen and was a bit surprised that they didn't do that in the prep room. Karen and Jack would have joked their way through it, I'm sure. I didn't think about it at the time, but the shaving must have taken place after I was anesthetized. When the hair was growing out, progressing through that itchy, prickly stage, I was thinking of the only other time I'd had my "privates" shaved.

In 1972, Karen and I decided that I would have a vasectomy. We had a boy and a girl and thought that was enough. Not having to be concerned about birth control also had its attraction. We were living in Logan, Utah, where I was going to graduate school to get a Ph.D. in psychology. I called our physician and told him what I wanted. I should have anticipated his response, since I knew he was bound to be a Mormon—his last name was "Bishop," for crying out loud.

"How old are you?"

"Twenty-nine."

"How many children do you have?"

"Two."

"I'd like to talk you out of it."

"I didn't call you up to have you talk me out of it. We know what we want. I'll call someone else."

At this point, I figured this bias toward having large numbers of children was likely to be rampant in this small, overwhelmingly Latter Day Saints community. We were going back to Spokane for my 10-year high school reunion in a few months, so I could have the procedure done there. We knew that Karen's sister's husband, Clyde, had had a vasectomy a few years earlier in Spokane. I called Clyde, who gave me the name of Dr. Harvey Weitz.

We drove to Spokane in August and contacted Dr. Weitz, who had me come in for a pre-surgical consultation. At that time, he explained the procedure, paying special attention to the fact that he didn't just tie off the ends of the vas deferens, but cut a section of it out and then double-tied both ends. I scheduled an appointment, though I had some misgivings, since his office was in an old house set back from busy Sprague Avenue. When I walked up to the door, I felt a bit like I was sneaking into a back-alley abortion clinic.

Dr. Weitz had instructed me to shave my entire abdomen and groin area before coming in. The night before my surgery, we went out drinking with old friends. What else would a young guy do the night before his vasectomy? We stayed out late, and I remember lots of razzing, comments related to the hope that the doctor was not drinking as much that night as we were. What are friends for, anyway? A bit hung over, I climbed into the tub at my mother-in-law's at 6 a.m. and very carefully shaved my nether region. Karen's mom wondered what I was doing in the bathtub so early, and for so long. Karen said I was shaving before my vasectomy, and then had to explain what a vasectomy was. Pearl had been raised at a time when such things were just not discussed.

Dr. Weitz was a nice enough fellow, and I did not seem to have post-surgical problems and have either been sterile or phenomenally lucky over the next several decades. He did, though, have sort of an odd bedside manner. The vasectomy is done under a local anesthetic, so I was cognizant of everything that was going on. I do not like to see gore and was happy that he provided me with neither a mirror nor a play-by-play analysis.

On the other hand, I was told the procedure was pretty much painless, so I didn't quite understand why he had to stretch my vas 37 feet into the adjoining room in order to excise the pieces.

He kept saying, "You're doin' fine, doin' fine." I kept saying, "Arrrrrgh. No I'm not, no I'm not."

Halfway through this ordeal, he stuck a syringe in front of my face with a bloody chunk of this little tube on the end of it, and said, "Looks just like a turkey quill, don't it?" A few years after we moved back to town, I read that his license to practice medicine was revoked by the state board because he had been playing fast and loose with prescribing narcotics. Thanks, Clyde. I owe ya one.

Over the years, there have been suggestions that having a vasectomy increases your chances of having prostate cancer. Research has not confirmed any such correlation. All the more reason to recommend vasectomies. The recovery from this outpatient procedure is swift: you walk funny for a few days, which gives your erstwhile friends who have gone through the procedure lots of laughs. The birth control benefit is virtually foolproof, and the lack of worrying about unwanted pregnancy is a huge relief to you and your partner. True, you should consider that the resulting sterility is going to be permanent, but I have one good friend who, after remarrying a younger woman, fathered a child after micro-surgery to reverse the procedure.

Previous Hospital Experience

My prior experiences as a patient in a hospital were for a tonsillectomy as a toddler, for polio at age 6, and for an angiogram and an attempted ablation of cardiac cells to control my ventricular tachycardia when I was 48. I have little memory of the tonsillectomy, so can't be sure if it bothered me much or not.

I do, however, have a few crystal-clear memories of my two weeks in the hospital with polio. I did not know that I had the disease until I was on my way home. I remember sitting in the back seat as we passed children playing in a park near downtown Salt Lake City. I announced to my parents that all the other kids on my ward had had polio. I remember being surprised and a little confused when they said that I did, too.

The first night in the hospital, they performed two spinal taps to confirm the polio diagnosis. Though I have only a vague recollection of the procedures, they were said to be very painful. What else would you expect when they jab a needle in your spine? On each occasion, Dad gave me a half dollar and told me to squeeze it hard while the spinal tap was being done. He must have been searching his brain for some way to help me through the ordeal. While it's true that tensing up can make an experience more painful, distraction is a proven technique for pain control. It seems to me that Dad's strategy, whether it was his intention or not, might have functioned as a way to give me some sense of control in a situation where none of us had much control over anything.

Thirty-five years later, I learned that Dad had carried those two coins in his wallet every day since I was in the hospital. They were so tarnished that they were almost black when he gave them to me when I was in my early 40s. They have been a treasure to me ever since. I had been keeping them on the top of my dresser, until we had a home burglary in the mid-1990s.

Several teenagers had broken into our house when we were away for a few days that winter. Among the missing items were the two half-dollars. I experienced the usual sense of violation and was angry about the things stolen, but nothing taken was as upsetting as the loss of those half dollars.

Several years later, on Dad's birthday, I was rummaging through my sock drawer and heard a clink. The coins were hidden inside a rolled-up pair of socks. I yelled out, "Yes!" and began to cry. I immediately called Mom and Dad and related to them the present I had just received on his birthday. I hope that he understood what those coins meant to me.

I wrote the following poem relating to my memories of that hospital experience. I know it's not about prostate cancer, but what the heck. The poem is another example of writing about difficult experiences, and I like it. My brother, Kerry, who always has nice things to say about my writing, says that it is his favorite.

OLFACTORY MEMORY

The smell of warm,
wet wool still
evokes the room
in the isolation ward
where they treated
kids with polio in 1950
by swathing their
skinny legs in
damp, heated blankets.

I'll bet the evidence
for the efficacy of
that therapy was

equal to that of
the olive-oil-on-my-
six-year-old-forehead
blessing of the Mormon elders.

My complete recovery
was more likely
due to luck or
maybe
the unyielding love of
my terrified parents or

maybe
outrage that my green

stuffed dog and
stack of comic books
were quarantined
when I left or

maybe
some nascent defiance
sparked by a nurse
sorely in need of an
occupational change
who forced me to drink
V-8 and eat mashed
canned sugar peas and
called me a baby when
I wet the bed (bitch).

March 6, 2009[4]

I remember feeling pretty spunky after a couple of days in the hospital, so aside from being homesick, having one cruel nurse, and being forced to leave behind my treasures when I went home, I tolerated the hospital stay fairly well.

Being hospitalized has proven to be much more difficult for me after I grew up. To get a glimpse of my reactions as an adult to being in the hospital, picture this. I'm lying in a room on the cardiac ward with Karen standing by my bed. She has been running back and forth from her new job as the Lilac Bloomsday Association Race Coordinator. It's only a few weeks until her debut at the head of this 12 Km run involving over 50,000 runners, so she's already under a ton of stress. Then she has to deal with people sticking things up my groin and into my heart. They have delayed the angiogram because I have

[4] Previously published in the 2009 issue of *Blood and Thunder: Musings on the Art of Medicine.*

had a migraine, but the headache has abated just in time, so the angiogram proceeds.

The nurse walks in. "We're ready to take you now."

My entire body immediately begins to tremble hard enough to shake the bed. Karen squeezes my hand.

"It will be okay," she says.

They wheel me through the halls. I have no idea why they do that with you lying flat on your back. Staring at the ceiling as it whizzes by contributes to a sense of unreality, anxiety, and loss of control. At least, that's what it does for me. But I don't like to go on carnival rides either, so maybe others don't mind. It seems as though it would be less upsetting if they left you sitting up until you got to your destination.

I'm now in a brilliantly lit room with stainless steel everywhere I look. There are various unfamiliar machines above me and video monitors to the side. A female technician leans over my quaking form.

"Are you cold? I'll get you a blanket."

"Hell no, I'm not cold. I'm scared."

"Oh, didn't they give you anything for that? We usually give Valium® back in the room. I'll put some in the IV."

From that point on, my memory is fuzzy, undoubtedly from the Versed®, which they've also added to the IV. Versed® is a narcotic drug noted for its amnesic properties. I do remember the warm rush that they told me to expect when they injected the contrast dye. I thought for sure that I had urinated, but they assured me that I had not. I remember much later telling them that they needed to hold on a minute and give me a bedpan because I did have to pee. I have another clear memory of watching the monitor and seeing the catheter snaking around inside my heart and coronary arteries (I think that's where it was).

The tranquilizing drugs were effective, because I do not recall any anxiety at the time. On the other hand, right now, I do feel anxious just thinking about that mental picture. I'm far different from my psychologist friend, Rob, who performed a mock sneeze during his angiogram. The medical people sort of freaked. He told them he did it because he had heard that your heart stopped when you sneezed, and he wanted to see if that was true.

Of course, he's the same guy who told me he took a suicidal client rock-climbing, got him positioned on a ledge, and yelled, "Go ahead and jump!" The guy apparently decided he wasn't so interested in killing himself, after all. I assume Rob's malpractice insurance was paid up. I can't see myself employing that therapeutic technique with a suicidal client. Rob's a great guy, but he still wonders why I refuse to accept his kind offer of flying with him in his home-made airplane.

I had no problem admitting my fear. After all, someone was going to be threading a catheter up through my groin all the way to my heart. One false move and an artery or the walls of the heart itself could be punctured. Or a mistake with the drugs could leave me brain damaged or dead.

Ultrarunning With the Arrhythmia

The day after my angiogram, I heard about a rumor that I was in the hospital following a heart attack. I regularly wrote articles and race reports for *Running Briefs*, the newsletter of the Bloomsday Road Runners Club, so that seemed like a good place to squelch the rumor. I submitted a poem about the angiogram, along with an article entitled "Psychologist Gets Whacked in the Head with a Two-by-Four." That's what it felt like. Long-distance running had been a central part of my life for 15 years. It provided me with a level of fitness I had not approached as a high school basketball player, let alone as an adult. I gained non-pharmaceutical stress relief and a combination of solitude and camaraderie. Running was now a large part of our social life.

I had completed the first 10 runnings of the Le Grizz 50 Mile Ultramarathon before I developed the arrhythmia. I ran the next 17 of them on anti-arrhythmic beta-blocker drugs. Considering my past history of childhood polio and rheumatic fever, I have always considered myself lucky to be able to be so active.

Whether it was denial or defiance, within a year after my diagnosis, I took on a running pseudonym. I had enjoyed Ivan Doig's *Winter Brothers* (1982). In this book, Doig retraced the travels along the northwest coast of the United States chronicled in the voluminous diaries kept by James Earl Swan throughout the middle of the 19th century. At one point, Swan is told by a Makah Indian friend that he has a "skookum tumtum," a "strong heart," because he sleeps with his door open and is not afraid of the spirits of the night. I combined those two words into one, "Skookumtumtum," and have since that time registered in all my races under that bastardized Native American name.

I think it's pretty funny that a number of ultrarunners appear to have forgotten my given name, but they can tell you who Skookumtumtum is. This goofy name may represent a healthy insistence, an optimistic view. Or maybe by focusing on heart strength when I had a heart problem, I was using denial to cope with my disease, thus proving once again that psychologists are susceptible to the same defenses as anyone else. I choose to view it as healthy optimism.

I had no way of knowing what would transpire 10 years later when I finished my 20th consecutive Le Grizz.

I invited my children and grandchildren to crew for me that day. It was a lot to ask. I am grateful that they traveled to the far northwest corner of Montana to support me. Karen and I rented a motor home so that we could all camp near the start at Spotted Bear. I had a difficult day, but finally finished, accompanied across the finish line by Karen, Steven, Sue, Heather, Dwain, Kaitlyn, McKenzie, and Rusty the dog. I knew that I was going to be given a special award. Travel with me now to the far northwest corner of Montana.

The shadows are lengthening at the Lion Lake picnic area that serves as the finish of the run. I don some warmer clothes, eat some chicken and jo-jo potatoes, and drink a beer. Race director Pat Caffrey, a giant of man you immediately know hails from Montana, tells me to get back to his truck near the finish as soon as possible, because my ceremony will be the first order of business before he hands out the other awards.

When we have all gathered, Pat says, "We have wanted to extend our connection to the Native people, and this year Maynard Kicking Woman, an elder of the Blackfeet tribe, has driven over from Browning to conduct a First Nations naming ceremony for Skookumtumtum. He will be assisted today by two Boy Scouts from the Order of the Arrow. Steve also will receive our first 'Chief 10 Bears' award."

Maynard, long raven braids falling over his shoulders, forms a circle with me and the Scouts and talks of Blackfeet customs and his own quest for sobriety. He tells us of the importance of rituals, such as the giving of names. In the middle of his speech he breaks into a chant, singing, I assume, in Blackfoot. Wow, this is the real deal.

Maynard continues his chant for several minutes. The group of weary but happy runners and crew are spellbound as he says something close to, "I have decided to name you 'Kioapita' (*that's what it sounded like, anyway*), which stands for 'Eagle Bear.' In legend, Eagle Bear was a bear that went away, but kept coming back. And you have kept coming back here every year to finish this race 20 times. I admire your dedication, but I do wonder if you are just a little crazy." Maynard continues, "The next part of the ceremony will take place down on the shore of the lake."

Holy crap. I hope that Blackfeet rituals don't include full-body immersion baptism such as I endured with the Mormons at age 8, because I am still shivering from the weather and my depleted state.

Maynard lights a length of sweetgrass and waves the smoke all over my body while continuing a new chant. His song becomes a haunting wail. We finish with me still on dry land. I am aglow looking at the faces of my family and this group of friends whom I have known and run with for a couple of decades.

Since I did not have a spelling of the Blackfoot name, I emailed Pat a few weeks later to find out how to write it out. He responded that Maynard said the name didn't spell out in English. Later, Pat wrote, "The actual spelling of Eagle Bear is Tiita Kiyo, pronounced Bee'-tuh Kyi-yo. The literal translation of Kiyo Tiita: Bear like an eagle." I don't suppose it matters. Even though I can no longer run long distances, I do have an authentic Blackfoot name and it is Eagle Bear. (Note: the tribe is "Blackfeet": the language is "Blackfoot.")

I have yet to dream up a creative name such as Skookumtumtum or Kiowa pita or Kiyo Tiita to help me cope with prostate cancer. Upon hearing this, those who know me well will probably breathe sighs of relief, since any name I concocted in this context could very well be unfit for polite company.

I now have several friends who have joined me as Chiefs by completing 20 Le Grizz runs. I'll tell you a story to give you an idea of the importance which ultrarunners can place on such milestones. A good friend of mine completed his 19th Le Grizz a few years ago in October. In the following spring, he was diagnosed with prostate cancer. He opted for brachytherapy, traveling from Montana to Seattle to have the radioactive seeds implanted. The first thing he asked the doctor before he agreed to the procedure was whether or not he would recover in time to get his training completed for Le Grizz in the fall. The doctor assured him that he'd have plenty of time

Five weeks before the Le Grizz run, he showed up at The Uncle Joe 50 Km Ultramarathon that Karen and I organized to raise funds for a scholarship that we award. He ran our race wearing a T-shirt that had pictures of 20 grizzly bears on it. Nineteen of the bears were in color. The last one was black and white, to be colored in upon his twentieth finish. That October, he finished number 20 with a beaming smile.

Again, I am reminded of the possible relationship between extreme exercise, free radicals, and prostate cancer. Sounds like a great subject for a research grant. For me, I guess it doesn't matter now one way or the other. I'm done with anything that even approaches "extreme" when it comes to exercise, and I am doing just about everything else I have heard about that boosts the immune system, so it can counter the effects of free radicals. So, before I start obsessing about what I might have done better, I'll refer again to my poem, "Assigning Blame," and move forward with a minimum of regret.

In the fall of 2010, I did not enter Le Grizz, but I had the distinct pleasure of filling in for Maynard to induct our friend, Mary Ann Clute, into the Chief Ten Bears group. Maynard was the emcee for a powwow that weekend, but gave me the information I needed to conduct a ceremony to rechristen Mary Ann as "Coyote Woman" in honor of being the first woman to complete 20 Le Grizz runs. I must note that one of Mary Ann's completions was accomplished while she was recovering from a procedure to destroy her thyroid gland. She's tough.

In 2010, Karen and I also worked at the Le Grizz finish line, which was not only a hell of a lot less effort, but also provided more opportunity to visit with runners and their crews. I felt much less devastated to miss out on running than I would have predicted just a few years ago. Maybe aging does bring a modicum of acceptance.

Inevitable Existential Questions

I imagine few people approach surgery for cancer without spending some extra time contemplating their mortality. It's said that such a focus often leads to the foxhole Christian response. I did not notice a significant change in my agnosticism after either my cardiac problems or my diagnosis of prostate cancer. I appreciated the kind intentions of my Christian friends when they prayed for me, but the notion of a personal God who involves Himself or Herself in the daily life of humans remains an unlikely, even absurd, notion to me. In 2007, I expressed this irreverent view in a poem.

POOP OCCURS

What I want
matters not,
except to Me and Mine.
No skyhook Father
strains to hear
my kneeling plea,

concerns himself
with how I am.

I Am, that's all.

The neutral Universe
has no care
for any whims of mine
or if I'm good or bad
or glad or sad.

It has its rules
that say
that X makes Y
with maybe help
from A or B.

Whatever is, Is.

October 12, 2007

The view expressed in this poem eliminates anguish
about what a person may have done morally wrong to
deserve cancer or to suffer other difficulties in life. Such a
world-view also simplifies things for me. I don't have to
try to reconcile the notion of a loving, omniscient, and all-
powerful Supreme Being with the presence of tragedy and
evil in the world. If He or She is all-knowing, all-
powerful, and loving, how could He or She let terrible
things happen to good people? Think childhood cancer,
Katrina, the Holocaust, children left without parents, and
sexual abuse.

This view also removes the question of a Being who
would let good things happen to evil people who mug,
molest, maim, and murder, or who allows the well-being
of the greedy bastards who rule the world. Lordy, Lordy,
The Reverend Pat Robertson and Rush Limbaugh are still

walking around fat and happy, and Dick Cheney is still sucking in oxygen despite a great deal of heart disease. Though I enjoyed Harold Kushner's book *When Bad Things Happen to Good People* (1981), even his more sensible attack on this problem didn't quite work for me. A lack of theistic belief eliminates a search for sins for which a person is being punished by way of a disease such as cancer. However, it does not eliminate questions about whether or not we bear some responsibility for our health status because of our lifestyle choices. How we live does influence our health, as I will discuss in detail in the FOLLOW UP chapter.

I best fit in the agnostic camp, which means that I don't really know if there is some sort of God or not. I also would place myself toward the atheistic end of that spectrum. "Poop Occurs" is, of course, an atheistic poem. Many of my readers will be people of faith. When they read "Poop Occurs" and the paragraph that follows, some people will have the urge to save me. Others will view the religious beliefs of others in a way similar to that of my friend, Dennis Clute, who says, "Whatever floats your boat." Some of the faithful will be appalled and dismiss anything else I have to say.

Regardless of your religious orientation, I hope you will look past any differences we may have in terms of belief and learn to use the other parts of this book, which deal with coping with a disease that strikes people of all faiths, and those of no faith. In fact, this brief detour into theology may prompt some of you to write a poem or short essay about how your own faith contributes to your being able to handle your disease or how your disease has challenged your faith. I encourage you to try your hand at this sort of writing. You might find it just as useful for you as writing that poem was for me.

Post-Surgery Hospital Stay

As you can tell by now, I am one of those people who has a difficult time being in the hospital. Before my prostate surgery, I told Dr. Golden about the one time I had a full-blown panic attack. Imagine the scene: It is pitch black, and Karen and I and the kids are sleeping in our small cab-over camper on the back of our Datsun pickup. Sullivan Lake is a gorgeous setting, and we are just up the road along Noisy Creek.

Out of the blue, I blast awake from a sound sleep, heart pounding and body shaking, desperate to jump out of the sleeping bag and out of the tight quarters of the camper. It takes me a moment to realize what is happening. *So this is what my clients talk about when they describe the terrors of their panic attacks. That's all it is, a panic attack, a false alarm. I'm okay. I can handle it. I just need to stay here and breathe till it's over*

I wait without awakening anyone, and the panic ends. I've done a good job calming myself with rational self-talk. But 30 years later, I haven't forgotten the experience.

When I was lying in my hospital bed waiting for my angiogram in 1992, I was feeling claustrophobic, on the verge of having a panic attack. A few times during the day before the procedure, it was all I could do to keep from ripping out the IV line and running out of the hospital. I was again fearful before my prostatectomy. This time, I decided to make things easy on myself. I talked to Dr. Golden and asked to have an order for Xanax® available in case I wanted it in the hospital.

I hope that you get the message in this book that making things as good as possible for yourself when you are confronting these sorts of scary issues is not only highly recommended, but commendable.

After surgery, I was in a lot of pain from spasms in my neck. I assumed the IV they placed there was the source of this problem. It wasn't until the second day after surgery that my complaints about my IV were successful in getting an IV nurse to move the line. She was able to use a vein in my bicep, but by then, stiffness and spasming had set up shop in my neck. I tried muscle relaxers, and Karen brought me a rice bag we heat in the microwave for sore muscles. I battled the nurses, who refused to heat the rice bag sufficiently to do me any good. They insisted on wrapping it in a towel. Of course, as soon as they left the room, I threw the towel on the floor. This problem caused a great deal of distress for nearly a week, but at least at home I could have the rice bag as hot as I wanted it.

Friends, Friends, Priceless Friends—In the first few days after surgery, I had a number of good friends stop by the hospital to commiserate or roast me with sarcastic humor. My sister and brother and the kids called from out of town, eager to see how I was doing. I suppose feeling cared for and being reminded of your good fortune to have so many close connections is one benefit of surgery.

At one point, a smiling face that transported me back a half-century appeared above the inflatable pressure socks at the foot of my bed. Todd Gee, oldest son of my closest high school friend, Mike, is, as they say, the spittin' image of his dad. I always enjoy talking with Todd. I'd had almost no contact with Mike since the mid 60s, as he moved around the country in a high-powered radio and TV career. A few weeks after my surgery, Mike phoned to see how I was doing, a welcome surprise.

Ron and Jane McDonald showed up, and Bill Greene dropped by when he was on call at the hospital. Bill later brought his wife, Linda, in to visit, as well. Bill's calm, confident presence buoyed me, just as it had when he supported me in the early days of my arrhythmia. Ginger kept checking in.

I mentioned my private practice partner, Dick Groesbeck, in the first chapter. Like Jack and Bill, he is my brother. I had talked with him about my upcoming surgery and knew he'd call to be kept abreast of my progress. The entire state of Washington was blanketed by a heavy snowstorm while I was in the hospital. The last thing I expected was for Dick to peer around the curtain after a treacherous 8 ½ hour drive over Snoqualmie Pass. Though I still wasn't in much of a laughing mood, his rude, crude, sarcastic banter had its predictable salutary effect.

The Verdict—As previously mentioned, during staging of prostate cancer, estimates are made about the aggressiveness of the disease based on PSA levels, the rectal exam, and the biopsy. Once removed, the prostate is microscopically examined in the lab. This more direct evaluation often leads to an upgrading of the severity of the disease. According to Ellsworth et al. (2003, page 99), "Approximately, 20 percent to 60 percent of men undergoing prostatectomy have a higher stage of prostate cancer when the pathologist reviews the surgical report."

My world was still bleary when Dr. Golden came in with the final pathology report. I recall that Dick was in the room, and Karen was on her way in to town from the Valley. I remember Dr. Golden drawing a diagram of my prostate positioned below the bladder, surrounding the urethra with the urethra poking out the bottom on its journey to the outside world. (I thought of using the title *A Urethra Runs Through It* for this book, but decided that Norman MacLean might be offended, and I doubted Brad Pitt and Tom Skerrit would be available for the movie version.)

Margins—The critical part of Dr. Golden's drawing showed little black marks on the right edge of the prostate with the label "positive margin." I remember my friend

Bert saying, "Negative margins, negative margins, that's what you really need to hear when they are done, negative margins." I was early in my research when I was talking to him about his prostatectomy, so I had to check on this notion of surgical margins.

A negative margin means that the pathologist observes space between the last cancer cells and the outside edge of the prostate tissue removed; thus, there are no malignant cells in this marginal area and, presumably, none in the adjacent tissue that remains inside the body. Conversely, a positive margin means there are cancer cells right up to the edge of the excised tissue, indicating a strong likelihood that more are lurking beyond that edge, ready to metastasize.

A few pages after their quote about the frequency of upgrading of staging upon final pathology, Ellsworth et al. note that ". . . in those with positive margins, there is an almost 50% chance that the PSA will increase within five years of surgery." And, of course, you don't want to see a non-zero PSA following surgery, since you no longer have a prostate to produce this antigen.

While it is true that there are some cells lining the urethra that produce tiny amounts of the PSA, having a PSA above zero after surgery usually means that there are some cancerous PSA cells roaming around someplace, with an unknown chance that they will end up somewhere, such as in your bones. That's when you are in a whole heap of trouble.

Dr. Golden indicated his surprise that I had a positive margin. "I didn't believe them. I went in and looked through the microscope myself—twice." And then he said something like, "I counted just a dozen or two dozen cancerous cells." The pathology report also noted that the cancer had penetrated the capsule that encircles the prostate. Another bad sign, but Dr. Golden remained optimistic. He said that I still had a 90 percent chance of my PSA never rising above zero.

<u>The Roommate</u>—When I arrived at my room after some time in the recovery room, I discovered that I had a roommate who also had undergone a prostatectomy a couple of days earlier. He talked incessantly, including graphic descriptions of his bladder spasms and the time he had yanked out his catheter with the balloon still inflated, blood flying everywhere. I never saw him because of the curtain between our beds, so I wouldn't recognize him if I met him on the street. As the hours and days passed, he entered into each conversation between me and my guests. At first I found him quite irritating. Soon though, reflecting on the love shown to me by my family and dear friends led me to change my view of my roommate:

PATIENT BECOMES PATIENT

His repeated intrusion
into my visitors' conversations
was wearing thin until
I realized I was going home
with the aid of
a friend who had driven
400 miles over snowy
mountain passes and
my dear Karen who'd
provide loving post-op care
that money could not buy
while he would be
schlepping his catheter bag
back to a one-man
apartment in a taxi.

February 5, 2009

In a sense, this poem is another example of managing emotion with self-talk. In there somewhere were thoughts such as, *This guy should shut up and quit bothering us. He is so rude. I shouldn't have to put up with his jabbering.* Before he left, I got myself to converse with him, which wasn't really a burden to me. I'm glad that I went through the process of viewing him differently. Not only did I stop being irritated and instead felt compassion, I also got another poem out of the deal.

I, too, wanted to be a good friend. Earlier I mention Roger Harman, a fellow retired psychologist who had been the teaching assistant in my first statistics class in 1965. In the late 1970s, Roger helped me train for my first marathon. We capped off our time by running the first 10 miles of the Coeur d'Alene Marathon together that year.

I had heard he was up in the cardiac ward following coronary artery bypass surgery. I was disappointed to find that my expectations of journeying to that ward were unrealistic. Up until the day I went home, I was unable to maintain my blood pressure when I stood up. I could barely walk to the bathroom without passing out, so a trip upstairs was out of the question. I'd had a similar reaction in 1992 when I had an angiogram. That time, I had to remain in the hospital overnight for what was supposed to be a same-day procedure. Remember, I'm also the guy who passes out when blood is drawn. That's just how my body responds to certain stressors, I guess.

Tom Dukich is one of the funniest people I have met, and he may be the most creative. He has a Ph.D. in psychology, but his first loves are art and music. Sometimes he combines the different disciplines to come up with some of the most thought-provoking, entertaining, zany and bizarre works around. His creations include my favorite, "Wunderkat," a perpetual motion machine combining two eternal truths: Cats dropped out of windows always land on their feet, and toast that falls off the counter always lands jelly-side down. You get the idea. I heartily recommend that you visit his website, www.tomdukich.com.

He and his art teacher/wife, Carolyn, once sent me a beautifully framed photo of a statue of a priest who had a large nose. Attached was a label that said "Bishop Steve." When they had seen the statue in a museum in France, they were so convinced it looked like me, they thought that I deserved the photo. Tom and Carolyn showed up at the hospital a couple of days after my surgery. I felt fortunate not to have ruptured my stitches from laughing while they were there. The following verse, including its intentional grammatical errors, will give you a good picture of what a hospital visit from the Dukiches is like.

FIRST SHOWER

My hospital bed was
triangled by wife Karen
plus Tom and Carolyn on
post-prostatectomy Day One
when she appeared,
a 20-something blonde whose
stunning beauty blended
my granddaughters,
daughter and wife.
Her "When they leave,
I'll help you with your shower"
upraised the six eyebrows before me.

When she was gone,
 I sotto-vocéd,
"Well, looks like this
will be the first test of
the 'nerve-sparing' surgery."

The comely creature
later stood by as they departed,
unfazed by Carolyn's
eye-batting farewell,
"Enjoy your baaaaath."

We showered; alas,
the only noteworthy blood-pooling
must have been in my legs
for I was so "shocky" I had
to sit with my head below my
knees on my way back to bed.

My erstwhile friends sent
a card from "Chief Nurse Sister Helga"
relaying complaints about
shower behavior "inconsistent with
the mission of this hospital."

Bless them.

Here is a replication of the inside of their get well
card, including the idiosyncratic grammatical style of
Sister Helga.

To: Mr. R. Steven Heaps
Fr: Chief Nurse Sister Helga
Re: Inappropriate shower manners

The little blonde nurse that attended
to your "needs" in the shower has
reported behavior on your part that is
not consistent with the mission of
those who run this hospital, the
Sisters of Mercy Charity and Chastity.

In the future, we recommends that
you attend to your alleged "hygiene

needs" on your own, without the help
of any little blonde nurses. Attached
inside is a photo of how I attend to
said legitimate needs and advice that
you conduct yourself similarly.

Yours is Christ, Sister Helga

The front of the card had a photo of a chubby lady in
a one-piece bathing suit dumping a bucket of water over
her head. I assume that must have been Helga, attending
to her legitimate needs with the cold shower treatment of
yesteryear.

Social Support and Prostate Cancer

I had all these wonderful friends and family members
concerned about me. My good fortune to have such a
wealth of love from them, when compared to my
roommate's relative isolation, reminds me to comment on
the power of social support in the battle against cancer.

What does science have to say about social support
and cancer? As with many areas, the most research
appears to have been done with breast cancer patients. A
striking testimony to the importance of social support
came from work done by Vanderbilt-Ingram Cancer
Center professor Meira Eppelein (Eppelein et al. 2011),
with the Shanghai Breast Cancer Survivor Study in China.
Women with breast cancer who had the highest scores on
social well-being had a 48 percent reduction in the rate of
cancer recurrence and a 38 percent lesser chance of dying
than those reporting the lowest levels of social well-being.

Another Internet post described a study (Stone, 1999)
which found that both high stress levels and low levels of
social support are correlated with significant increases in
the probability of having abnormally high PSA scores.
These results are intriguing. However, correlation does

not prove causation. Other variables, such as unhealthy eating and drinking patterns, which may accompany both low levels of social support and elevated stress, could be what matters.

Social support clearly has a beneficial effect on men's *adjustment* to having prostate cancer. Roberts, Lepore and Helgeson (2006) found that men's higher levels of social support measured soon after prostate cancer treatment were related to better mental functioning three months later. Their work indicated that this benefit in mental functioning occurs because social support helps the men to cognitively process the experience of having cancer. Through this processing, they end up with fewer intrusive thoughts and a lesser need to continue to search for meaning.

If Man as a species is nothing else, he is a social animal. It seems to me that the older we get, the more we focus on the importance of our relationships with others. Among all the deathbed regrets people suffer, it's my guess that thoughts of the quality of our relationships with those close to us are among the most painful. While anytime is a good time to nurture such relationships, when serious illness raises the likelihood of your dying sooner than you expected, such matters vault straight to the top of the priority list.

Let's assume that your illness has led you to spend time thinking about your social connections, and that you have decided to enhance this part of your life. To do so will probably require you to alter some aspects of your behavior. Suppose you carry a large load of resentment toward your father. He divorced your mom when you were 8 years old, and while he always made certain that your physical needs were satisfied and you had good visits every other weekend, your mom has spent the rest of her life alone and depressed. You also feel cheated out of having a "regular dad," as did your friends. Now he's old, and you have a serious illness, and you still resent him, and that resentment keeps you away from him. You have decided you want to decrease your resentment and increase your contact with the Seven Cs method.

Applying the Seven Cs

You can begin with the first part of the Seven Cs to counter the self-talk that fuels your resentment. It will then be easier to alter your actions so that they more in line with how you want to be.

So let's start with CATCH. Spend a few minutes thinking about your dad. Remind yourself to be aware of the thoughts that are rumbling around in your head.

Okay, now CALM yourself by closing your eyes and taking five slow deep breaths, while you think about your favorite place outdoors.

Feel better? Now you are ready to CREATE a list of the thoughts that make up your internal dialogue. What comes up? Maybe you get stuck with thoughts like *it isn't fair; I didn't have a dad like Fred next door, whose dad was home every night; my mom never recovered from the split, and he's just an asshole.* These are just some possibilities. Write down what comes up for you. Don't censor yourself; whatever is there is fine.

Time to work to CHALLENGE the items on your list. Take them one at a time. Ask yourself questions about the thoughts. For example, *Who said life would be fair? It is what it is. We just need to deal with it rather than wallow in self-pity. Is it really true that I didn't have a dad? We did have good times together. I need to remember that. Is he really just an asshole? Hey, he is a guy just like I am, who made mistakes and has good and bad points. He didn't try to hurt me. He was just trying to figure out how to live his life. Does Mom bear any responsibility? She had a rough time, but she made choices after he left and never got herself going. That's not completely his fault. Maybe I can still connect with him, and I'd probably be glad that I did.*

Next, CHOOSE from some options about what you can do to make things better. You might: (1) invite him for coffee, (2) call him to check in, (3) find things to ask him for advice about, (4) take the kids to his house and (5) stop by and ask if you could help him around the yard.

That's a good start. Now make certain you follow through. For example: *This week I'll invite him for coffee on Wednesday, and next week I'll take the kids over on the weekend. I'll COMMIT myself to continue to do one of those each week and add one or two of the other options after a couple of weeks.*

CONGRATULATE yourself for taking steps that will make your life richer.

Again, there are lots of things over which you are going to have little or no control while you deal with your disease. All the more reason to take charge of any things over which you can exert some control, especially if they are things that are beneficial to you anyway.

4

RECOVERY

Dick helped Karen haul me home before he made the wintry return trek across the Cascades to Bellingham. My memories of the trip from the hospital are pretty fuzzy, probably because I was still in significant pain in my neck from the spasms caused by the IV line. Hershey was at the door to greet me. He is used to Karen and me being around to take him for a walk a couple of times each day, so we were very grateful to Ron and Marie Challender and Ron and Jane McDonald, who came over on different mornings to slog through the deep snow with our big baby. Maybe their attention made it easier for him to refrain from repeating the performance described in the poem on the following page.

ORGANIC ALARM

First it's the jangling shake
of licenses and rabies tags,
then a cold nose under the covers,
briefly rebuffed but returning
with the persistence of a
cookie-seeking toddler.

It escalates to a four-footed slither,
paw after paw up and
over one of us to flop in between,
95 pounds of
squirming canine slobber,
95 pounds of
still-puppy flesh,
a baby with limbs flailing
under a twirling mobile.

Licking and nipping, nipping
and wriggling and licking, he's
finally pushed off for one last
respite before an encore
performance forces us up to
feed the dog and meet the day.

July 7, 2008

On the second or third day home, Karen had run out to
the store, and I was feeling very shaky and vulnerable. I had
been teary all day. Maybe because I was alone for the first
time, or because of some long-lingering after-effects of the
anesthesia, or stress from the surgery, but at any rate I was
extremely anxious. I phoned my friend, Dick.[5] I am

---

[5] I cannot resist telling you that when Karen read an early draft of this
section, I could hear her laughing in the family room. She came into
the office where I was working on the computer, and she said, "I

fortunate to have friends with whom I feel comfortable sharing just about everything that is going on with me, even reactions that many men would see as pretty wimpy. Luckily, he was home, and I rambled on through my crying about how frightened I was, how vulnerable I felt, blah, blah, blah. I have no recall of what he said, but, as usual, it was useful for me to talk with him.

The Catheter

You can't talk about prostate surgery without talking about catheters. I did appreciate the fact that this very necessary device was installed while I was anesthetized. In fact, when I wrote the last sentence, I unknowingly crossed my legs! Like most guys with whom I've talked, I dreaded walking around with the end of that thing trailing out of my wingwang. When you are in the hospital, the tube is attached to a large collection bag that is pinned to the side of the bed. To walk around, you are given the option of using a small bag that straps to your leg. I know men who switched to the small bag frequently, even going to stores and to work with it. I guess they might have pretended that it was an ankle holster for a nine-millimeter Glock to help them get through the day. I chose to stay in the house for the two weeks until the catheter was removed, and I rarely used the small bag.

I think that being tethered to the catheter for two weeks was a major factor in my sense of helplessness and vulnerability. And you **ARE** vulnerable. What if the damn thing got yanked? What if you stepped on it? Remember

---

think you left out the word 'friend' in this sentence." Somehow, I had indeed typed the sentence, "I phoned my Dick." It was one of those times where the more one person laughs, the more the other laughs, until you're not sure if you are laughing about the joke or laughing about the laughing. We did decide that, with this being about the prostate and all, Sigmund Freud was alive and well.

Hershey and the hide-a-bed? I spent way too much energy worrying about Hershey doing his usual "so what if I weigh 95 pounds; I am, indeed, a lap-dog" routine. I wasn't very successful at ignoring the vivid images of him ripping out my stitches and puncturing the urine bag, or yanking out the catheter so that the inflated balloon on the end reamed my urethra out to the diameter of the Holland Tunnel.

In fact, Hershey was such a good boy that he never tried to climb up on me. He sat next to the bed or couch, licked my hand, and reveled in being petted. He never got near the catheter or bag. Also, I had no problem climbing the stairs to the master bedroom, and we soon decided that moving the hide-a-bed into the family room had not been necessary after all. Bill and Karen returned it to the office.

I found sleeping with the catheter in place to be rather disconcerting. I worried again about whether I would be able to sleep, whether the damn thing would get tangled, come out, wake me up, and so on. I had to work with my own self-talk to calm down and view it as only a temporary nuisance. Of course, this meant saying things to myself such as, *It's okay. You have had lots of practice with relaxation training, and you can use what you know to help you drift off. There have been no reports in the paper of men becoming permanently entwined in their catheter hoses, so you will probably survive.* After I refocused with more reasonable ideas, I slept pretty well. Also, just sleeping in bed with Karen was reassuring to me. I'd had only a few nights in the previous 44 years when she had not been in bed with me. Yes, I still didn't like to have the catheter in me with the bag pinned to the sheet, but I didn't feel alone.

Later I thought of a brief way to talk about the catheter.

ANASTAMOSIS[6]

After you yank my prostate
you're going to
shove a WHAT?
up my WHERE?
until WHEN?

Sheesh.

February 5, 2009

Control and Acceptance—Finding a Balance
People who know me will point out that I do not like
to be cold. It can take me an hour of standing on the dock
before I can get myself to jump into the lake to swim.
Sometimes I never succeed in taking the leap. Even as a
child enthusiastic about any chance to swim, my teeth
chattered, and my lips literally turned blue when I got out
of a pool or lake.

One of my fondest childhood memories is of Dad
briskly rubbing my arms with a towel to warm me up
when I finished swimming. A few years ago, I had a near-
flashback experience when toweling my own arms after a
swim in a cold lake. I felt an immediate return to those
days, a sense of connection to Dad, and a nostalgic ache
to see him just one more time.

In bed or on the hide-a-bed or sofa, I could easily
stay warm with blankets and sometimes a warm rice-bag.
I found the heat very comforting. When it came to
showering, I came up with a plan that many would judge

---

[6] An anastamosis is the connection in which the ends of the urethra
have been sewed together after the prostate is removed. To prevent
urine from leaking into the abdominal cavity while the anastamosis
heals, a catheter is inserted to take urine directly from the bladder to
the outside world. Useful and clever, but a hassle, for sure.

as wimpy or silly, but I found it helpful. Karen and I had a showering ritual (yeah, I wish it was a ritual in which we both were in the water together, but that was a long way from my mind at that time). We have a small half-bath just off the family room—toilet, sink, and shower. Fifteen minutes or so before my shower, she would put a small portable heater in the room and leave it on high. By the time I entered the room, it must have been at least 90 degrees. I was not going to be any more uncomfortable than I had to be. In fact, I also insisted on keeping the heater running while I was in the shower. Looking back, it's clear to me that this is another example of my searching for something I could control and then doing so.

Locus of Control—In 1954, Julian Rotter formulated the notion of locus of control. A great deal of research followed, exploring the extent to which people believe that they can influence events in their lives by their behavior (having an "internal locus of control") versus believing that fate or some other outside force is the major determiner of what happens to them (having an "external locus of control").

The latter view leads to a much more passive stance. If everything that happens to you is due to factors outside of yourself, over which you have no say, a feeling of helplessness is a likely outcome, and you are likely to act as though you cannot affect your world. Why bother? The former stance, having an internal locus of control, results in a more proactive approach to life.

However, if an internal locus of control is only viewed through the rear-view mirror, it may lead people to blame themselves for their disease, if they think that their actions have caused it. A better strategy is to apply, in a forward-looking direction, a locus of control style that puts a reasonable amount of emphasis on how your own behavior can affect your health. Thus, rather than my castigating myself for not following up immediately when my PSA rose, I will be better off if I decide what I can do from this point on to improve my health. I can harness an internal locus of control oriented to the future to follow a healthy diet, for example.

Inspired by Rotter's work, Wallston and Wallston (1978) developed a locus of control scale that focuses specifically on medical issues—naming it, unsurprisingly, the Medical Locus of Control Scale. I spent a fair amount of time reading the literature in this area and came away with the sense that the relationship between scores on the Medical Locus of Control Scale and health-related behavior and outcomes had not been completely worked out.

Maybe that's just me—getting old and not doing enough research. I do know that elaborating on the details of the burgeoning research in this area is beyond what I want to do here. You can check out the state of this work on your own, if you so wish. What is important for my purposes is to remember that having an internal locus of control can reduce depression by helping protect us from developing the sort of learned helplessness previously discussed in the DECISION chapter.

A view of ourselves and the world that revolves around an internal locus of control must be realistically married to a recognition of the limitations of the degree to which we have control over our health. We need to accept the fact that there are a number of factors that affect our health that are unrelated to our actions—factors over which we do not have much, if any, control.

Acceptance—Thus, like many things in life, a balance of forces is important. Acceptance of things as they are is the opposite of seeking to exert Control over the world. Acceptance is an absence of demanding that the world be different than it is. An acceptance of reality is valuable in managing one's life. Often, people get so caught up in denial or in focusing on how they think things ought to be, that they get frozen, paralyzed, and fail to take the sorts of actions that they can take to move forward.

I recently watched again one of my favorite movies, *Sometimes a Great Notion*, based on the Ken Kesey novel with the same title. Henry Fonda plays Henry Stamper, the monumentally cantankerous patriarch of a logging family caught in a battle with the local union. His ungrammatical motto, "Never Give a Inch," is carved into a cross section of a Douglas fir nailed to the living room wall. In conversation, the family slogan predictably becomes, "Never Give a Goddamn Inch."

Henry dies after losing his arm when a tree falls on it. In the movie's final scene, his son, Hank (Paul Newman), preserves the uncompromising family attitude by towing a four-raft train of logs down the river with Henry's arm lashed to the top of a pole, the fingers positioned to present a single-digit bird salute to the incensed union members on the shore.

I was thinking that the idea of never giving an inch may border on too much denial with regard to cancer, so I decided I'd adopt a mantra or motto of "Never Give a Foot, a Yard, or a Goddamn Meter." After all, a modicum of stubbornness in the face of disease may actually pay off.

John Gottman, a psychologist specializing in treating couples, found that his earlier methods, focusing on change and control, helped about one out of every two couples with whom he dealt. While that was hopeful, Gottman wanted to be even more effective. In his early work, he taught couples to make changes in their behaviors that were more supportive of their relationships. In his revised protocol, he added components which helped each person to accept things about their partner that bothered them, rather than to demand out loud or in their internal self-talk that their partner be how they wanted them to be. Obviously, he did not encourage them to accept such things as abusive behavior. With the addition of these acceptance strategies to the control techniques in his expanded protocol, many additional couples benefited (Gottman, 1994).

Steven Hayes of the University of Nevada at Reno has built an extremely helpful therapeutic model called Acceptance and Commitment Therapy, which combines these two forces. Briefly, people are taught to accept, rather than to bemoan, the reality of their current world and to commit themselves to taking charge of behaviors through which they can make step-by-step improvements in their lives. This school of thought counters helplessness by promoting the sorts of actions that can be taken, without denial of the way the world actually is.

With these ideas in mind, regardless of what treatment you choose for prostate cancer, I encourage you to take control of every small thing that you can. Take control of what you can do, especially if taking control of something makes you feel less helpless and helps you cope with the situation.

The time will come when you have done all you can do to control the outcome. You've done your research in books, journals, and on the Internet; you've consulted and gotten second and maybe even third opinions; you've talked to others who've had various forms of treatment, and you've chosen a treatment plan that seems best for you. At this point, you can feel confident that you have done what you could to understand and control the relevant factors outside of you. It is time to let go, to accept the reality of where you are.

When you have reached the point at which there is little you can do to control what is happening with your disease, never forget that you are always left with control of your own emotions and behavior. You can choose to be kind, to be curious, to be active. You can commit yourself right now to begin to use the self-control methods described in this book, to help you replace the dysfunctional thoughts and emotions that detract from the quality of your days, and to take charge of behaviors that can improve your satisfaction with your life experience.

As for my own life, I am going to continue to find things that I can do despite my disease, without ignoring or denying the reality of my cancer in a way that might lead me, say, to neglect to get my PSA checked at appropriate times, or to refuse to make informed decisions about treatment.

In concluding this discussion of control versus letting go, I must point out that none of these ideas are completely new. In fact, if you put the notion of truly accepting rather than fighting the reality that you face, and add that to taking control of whatever you can actually control, you end up with The Serenity Prayer of Alcoholics Anonymous, don't you? If I were a scholar of the Bible or other antiquities, I could probably quote much earlier examples, too. Feel free to do so. Send me the results of your search.

A Detour into Heart Surgery

I did enough of these things to prepare before my prostate surgery that I was confident I'd done everything I could do. It was time to leave the rest of it to the skill of the surgeon and his team. Two years later, I found myself going through a similar process, this time dealing with my heart. Heart? Aren't you a friggin' ultramarathoner? I know, I know.

As I said before, I've always known how fortunate I have been to be able to run and be active. Along with my history of polio, I also had rheumatic fever twice, at ages 3 and 8. The first time, I was in bed for a year. Family lore was that I had to learn to walk all over again afterward.

I have almost no memory of that time. I do remember my sister, Lynne, hauling me around the neighborhood in a wagon when she probably had more enjoyable things to do. I also know that for decades, Mom, who was 5 foot 2 inches tall and not much over 100 pounds, would flex her biceps to show people the muscles she had developed from carrying me around that year. That must have been scary for her and Dad. I was lucky to have parents who took such good care of me.

For the past several years, my mitral valve had been leaking more and more, until I arrived at the point at which surgery to repair it was recommended. In the past, cardiologists recommended delaying surgery until the leaking (also called regurgitation) produced significant symptoms. With this strategy, by the time surgery was performed, patients were short of breath with little exertion, or had developed significant pulmonary hypertension and an enlarged heart. More recently, the recommendation has been to take advantage of the window of opportunity during which the valve shows considerable regurgitation, but before the damage to the heart has progressed. This strategy has produced better success in repairing mitral valves, rather than having to replace them with mechanical, pig, or cow valves. I decided to follow the recommended treatment.

It seemed quite odd to be agreeing to heart surgery when I was not experiencing any great difficulties. It's just plain weird to have someone cutting into your heart when you don't feel sick. Now that I think about it, it's pretty weird to ever have someone cutting into your heart—period. When they are doing so while sitting 20 feet away at a computer terminal, operating a robot that they have tunneled in through your armpit, it reaches the surreal.

True, at last May's Lilac Bloomsday 12 Km run, I was frustrated that, despite doing some darn good training (for an old guy), it seemed that I never could really push myself as I had in the past; "no Go-Power" was how I termed it. I did, however, run fast enough to earn my second age-group medal in 31 attempts. I had a good summer of training for the Le Grizz 50 Mile Ultramarathon that I had completed for all 27 of its iterations.

In October on the day of that year's race, I did not feel overly confident, because a sudden cold snap had left us with zero degrees Fahrenheit at the start. Still, I had finished this race under difficult conditions in the past, including the year when I wrenched my back the day before, spent 24 hours in the bed of our camper passing a pee bottle out when necessary, then running bent over like someone with a severely twisted spinal cord. Maybe it was only (or mostly) the cold at the 28th Le Grizz, but I never could seem to get into a rhythm, and by 35 miles, I climbed into the truck and rode to the start. (Note to self: If you do that, you get to the finish line in time to drink a bunch of beer and feel well enough to visit with friends.)

Maybe, though, the regurgitation in my mitral valve made it just that much more difficult that, as I told people afterward, "For the first time, it just didn't seem to be that important to finish." Nonetheless, finishing Bloomsday under an hour at age 65 and dropping out of a 50-mile race at the 35-mile mark do not seem to be your usual signs of cardiac problems requiring surgery.

The explanations of the cardiologist and cardiac surgeon, and my independent reading, did not suggest that there was a variety of treatments from which to choose.

As with prostate cancer, I learned a great deal about the mitral valve problem and the surgery. As I think about how difficult and complicated the decision about treatment for prostate cancer seemed to be, the decision about the mitral valve surgery was quite straightforward. I don't remember having much, if any, fear of dying during or soon after the prostatectomy. Maybe because the valve repair involved my heart, rather than some weird little gland like the prostate that we rarely think about, I was concerned about dying from the heart surgery. Even the use of the robotic rather than the open-chest surgery required my being on the heart-lung bypass machine with my heart stopped for a couple of hours.

Before the surgery, I would think, *Shit, they are going to stop my heart; I hope they can restart it.* Silly, I know; they do this successfully all the time—it's routine for them. (Notice the attempt at rational, calming self-talk.) On the other hand, in my reading I noted that they said the mortality rate in the surgery was low. Then they said, "Two percent." Low, my butt. A tenth of a percent, that's what I call low—but two out of a hundred?

So I mentioned my concern to Dr. Siwek, the surgeon. His answer, later echoed in response to most questions I had for him, his physician's assistants, and the nurses, was, "Well, it's heart surgery. We aren't fooling around." He did tell me that his mortality rate was a third of a percent. That sounded much better. I could buy that as "low." Of course, I had to agree that this was heart surgery, and we weren't fooling around, which got me to thinking a great deal about the chances of my death occurring in the near future, rather in that vaguely imagined time sometime many years from now. This sort of thinking had several consequences; first, as I looked around, I had a renewed sense that all the "stuff" we owned was of little importance. All the things I especially valued, such as books, my running awards, the shotgun I received for Christmas at age 12, and my dad's shotgun which I inherited, will most likely be chucked out after I am gone, of no importance to anyone. This also is a time when it becomes clear that the opinions others may have of you, the need to have things be a particular way, and making mistakes all simply fade in importance.

A Novel Sort of Will—I have always been certain that it is the loved ones, the relationships, and the memories that matter in our lives. So, though I wished I had more time to write, edit, and rewrite, I got busy in the last few days before my heart surgery and worked on what I thought of as an emotional will. Karen and I each had a regular will drawn up by our attorney years ago to delineate what was to happen to our physical goods and financial assets. We also each signed a Durable Power of Attorney and a Living Will or Health Care Directive. A Living Will designates who was to make decisions about our medical treatment in the event that we were not capable of doing so, as well as the extent to which we would like treatment to be carried out when the likelihood of survival with some sort of quality of life was near zero.

This emotional will was something quite different. I had read about the idea in a couple of places, one in the unlikely location of a financial article that I have not been able to relocate. The idea of the emotional will is to write to significant others some thoughts that you would like to leave to them. This document can take any form you want. One may wish to offer thanks and appreciation, apologies and regrets, a recounting of meaningful times and events, wishes for the future, or some other valued messages.

So I did. I wrote a series of emotional wills. But hedging my bets, assuming I'd probably make it through the surgery, I didn't print the letters, but left the writing in a series of files on our computer where they'd be easy to edit later. I'm sure that, given time, I'll want to make changes, clean up the language, and add some things and subtract others. I wrote a message for my wife, my son and daughter and their spouses, my grandkids and my sister and brother. In our portable safe, where I expected my wife and kids would search soon after my death, I left a note asking them to print out each file and give it to the appropriate person.

Now, fortunately, I can go back and do whatever editing I want. I encourage you to complete such an exercise. You don't have to wait until you are facing a medical crisis. I think that most of our loved ones would treasure such a document after we are gone. Don't be surprised if this is an extremely emotional experience. In a way, you are practicing saying goodbye. I cried almost continuously as I wrote—of course, that's just me. I cry easily and frequently. You might breeze through the process unaffected (but I doubt it).

Here's one final example of unreasonable self-talk from *Behaving Well* that surprised Edmund Fantino. Even with all the proactive things he was doing to deal with having cancer, he noted that our behavior is not always consistent. His dentist told him that he was going to need a gold crown. Fantino's automatic thoughts centered on why spend the money, since he might soon be dead anyway. He quickly recognized that this sort of fatalistic thinking was not in his best interest and was able to put an end to it.

I must admit that I have had some brief thoughts similar to that. For example, when considering the heart surgery: *What if my PSA skyrocketed a few months after the surgery? Even worse, what if I then had metastasized disease to the bones? It would suck to endure the heart surgery if I were going to die before the valve problem was causing significant problems in my life. Why not just let it go?* Another couple of poems surfaced out of these thoughts and fears.

IN THE STILL OF THE NIGHT

When you learn
that the surgeon
is going to enter your
heart
to fix a leaky
valve,
you may
awaken
shaken
in the still of the night,
sleep
skewered
by questions
that have no answers.

December 5, 2009

A GIFT

They say my mitral valve
is broken,
flaps torn like some
bullet-ridden foe of
the Red Baron.
I guess I'll jump through
their "window of opportunity"
for a valve repair—
less oinkin' and mooin'
and clickety-clackin'
than a new valve.

Bill's running well
after his bypass;
he says now we'll
each have a new heart—
a Gift,
Magic.
I wonder if I can
match his attitude.

December 9, 2009

I did have the surgery. My mitral valve was successfully repaired, and my heart was successfully restarted after being on the bypass pump. The early part of recovery was made more difficult when my atrial fibrillation returned for a couple of weeks. Add that arrhythmia to a condition called atalectasis, in which your lungs don't re-inflate all the way and remain partially filled with fluid at the bottom, and you have the perfect recipe for the strange and scary experience of not being able to get your breath and not being able to lie down to sleep, because it feels like you are suffocating. I will forever look more compassionately on anyone walking around the grocery store with an oxygen bottle.

Though we did not know it at the time, while I was in the hospital, Karen developed shingles. She was in more and more pain over the first few days after I returned home. When she finally went to the doctor, the diagnosis was made. Shingles, while common, can be exceedingly painful, and she had a bad case that lasted for several months, despite treatment with the most effective medication available. A large proportion of the population carries the *varicella-zoster* virus, the chicken pox virus, in their bodies for years.

The disease appears to be precipitated by stress. No surprise that her condition began when it did. I'm not certain that I completely appreciated, at the time, what she was going through with the shingles added to her worries about me and her dedication to do everything she could to help me, but I do now. Food from the Greenes, and food plus an entire season of *Boston Legal* delivered by Ginger Metcalf, sustained us until the night that our daughter, Heather, surprised us by flying in from Portland to fill our hearts with her caring spirit and our freezer with vegetarian lasagna.

I resumed running, though after two years, I still walk on many days, and when I run, it is at a pitifully slower pace. Whereas I used to be one of the faster runners in my age group around Spokane, now even somewhat overweight ladies pass me on the Centennial Trail below our house. If nothing else, I have become even better at not taking things for granted. When I was thinking about the importance of humor and our well-being, the following line about valve and arrhythmia problems popped into my head: "It leaks, and it's got a short circuit, but it's the only pump I've got." You might see some movement toward acceptance there.

Continence? Well, It All "Depends"

I took the side trip into heart surgery while discussing the usefulness of balancing acceptance of the uncontrollable and taking control of what you can, indeed, control. Time to return to the prostate. An early recovery milestone is the removal of the dreaded catheter. One of my friends who'd had the surgery had told me, "The day they remove that catheter will be one of the best days of your life." Of course, he's also the guy who later told me that pomegranate juice was delicious—sure, if you supersaturate it with sugar. Then again, he drank his from freshly squeezed fruit on the streets of Tel Aviv.

At my two-week visit, Dr. Golden examined my incision and reassured me that the lumpy part in the middle was not a problem. He said it would smooth out over time. (In fact, it has, and the bright vermillion color has faded to a dull brown-red four years later.) Then he snipped off the side tube of the catheter, deflating the balloon inside my bladder. He said something about it briefly feeling odd when he pulled the tube out. Then, "Zoooooop," he quickly pulled the catheter out. Yep, it felt odd, but didn't hurt. He then stuck a stainless steel pan under my penis and said, "Okay, begin to urinate. Now stop the flow."

I was relieved that there was no pain. It wasn't until three years later that I heard from a friend that the removal of his catheter caused the most pain he had ever experienced in his life. I was pleased that at this first opportunity, I was able to have almost complete control over my urination. Maybe I wasn't going to be wearing Depends® for the rest of my life. I showed Dr. Golden the large diaper things we had purchased, and he laughed and said to put them away. He gave me some small pads to insert in my undershorts and said they'd do the trick. They did. I used the small pads for a couple of weeks and diligently completed my Kegel exercises.

Kegel exercises were invented in the 1950s by a physician named Arnold Kegel to help incontinent women. Kegels consist of tensing and relaxing muscles in the pelvic floor, called the pubococcygeus or PC muscles. Dr. Golden suggested that I start urinating, then stop it for a few seconds and repeat that several times. When doing Kegels, it is important not to involve the muscles of your buttocks, legs or abdomen. Think of having a strong urge to defecate or urinate and needing to hang on until you reach a toilet. Repeat the exercises five to ten times per day to improve urinary continence.

As with most exercises, it's not easy to continue to do Kegels on a consistent basis. For the six weeks prior to my surgery, I completed Kegels several times each day, along with the other exercises I was doing. This preparation may have been a factor in my quick recovery of continence. If you are still leaking months after your surgery, I suggest practicing Kegels daily. You might simply make a mark on your calendar each time you complete a set of Kegels. Check the calendar each night and aim for a goal of some number of marks per day.

You might wonder why all this is necessary. Why does taking the prostate out lead to incontinence in the first place? With an intact prostate, you have three things to aid you in urinating only when you wish to do so: the external sphincter, the sphincter at the neck of the bladder, and the prostate. After surgery, all that is left is the external sphincter. You have spent years not using this sphincter because the other two structures have pretty much taken care of business for you. Not surprisingly, your external sphincter may not be well developed.

Over time, I have gotten away from regularly doing Kegels. It would probably behoove me to do them more religiously, since I do occasionally leak a small amount, usually when I am running or immediately after finishing a run. If you happen to find your shorts getting wet when you are running, do what I do. Either ignore it, or, if you are in a race, splash some water down your front at the next aid station.

One day I stopped on a run to answer the questions of an elderly couple on the Centennial Trail that runs along the Spokane River below our house. After a few minutes I noticed that I had dripped enough on the ground that a wet spot was clearly visible. I decided that was probably a good time to continue my run. Fortunately, as previously mentioned, I am not easily embarrassed.

When one of my young friends ended up in the medical tent with heat stroke after the Bloomsday 12 Km run a few years ago, she told me she didn't drink fluids the previous night, in the morning, or during the run. She was afraid she would have to stop to pee at the porto-potties or wet her pants during the run. I took it upon myself to provide some fatherly advice, "Carol, if you want to be a Real Runner, just go ahead and pee in your shorts. Yes, there are tens of thousands of people around, but if you toss a cup of water down your front at an aid station, no one never will know. Plus, you can run faster without worrying about stopping."

If you are someone a bit more modest than I am, I suggest that for a while, at least, you stick one of those little pads in your shorts. If you like fiction, read some of Philip Roth's novels in which the protagonist has had a prostatectomy that left him incontinent and with erectile dysfunction. In *Exit Ghost* (2007), Nathan Zuckerman ruminates about the upcoming procedure, in which a catheter will be snaked through his urethra, to inject collagen where the bladder meets the urethra, to ameliorate his recalcitrant incontinence. Zuckerman's sense of shame over having "accidents" is a sad consequence of this problem.

While Roth exaggerates the rate of occurrence of serious problems with incontinence after modern prostatectomy surgery, the rest of the depiction of his character's reactions to the aftermath of his surgery suggests to me that Roth has probably had prostate cancer and opted for surgery. Of course, maybe his story rings so true just because he is a great novelist who has read about or listened to the experiences of others. Hey, I wonder if he'd read a draft of this book and give me some feedback. Nah, Pulitzer Prize winners probably don't do that sort of thing out of the goodness of their hearts. The good news is that the rate of incontinence after prostatectomy is now very low, in the 2 percent range.

Physicians are often in a hurry, and thus, may not take adequate time to ensure that we, up on the examination table, understand their instructions. Also, when we are receiving information from them, we may be in an emotional state that prevents us from retaining what they have said. Of course, sometimes we are timid about asking questions, and sometimes the doctor doesn't get around to covering all that needs to be covered.

It is likely that one of these factors was important for one friend that I talked to about his incontinence after his prostatectomy. He was not making improvement in accordance with what he had been led to expect. As we talked, I discovered that the Kegels he thought he was doing involved bearing down and squeezing the last drop of urine out as he finished voiding. I described the correct way to contract the PC muscle and sent him written instructions. He called a month or so later saying, "Everything is normal."

With incontinence and other issues, I urge you to take a paper and pen, a small audio recorder, or your wife or a friend with you to your doctor appointments to increase the chances that you will leave with a clear understanding of your condition, your treatment plan, and the things you need to do to help yourself. I try to always have a list of questions and concerns with me at any doctor visit. If I don't, I often find later that there was something I forgot to mention.

Once I had badly sprained my ankle on a hike along the ocean near Pt. Reyes, CA, the day after a 33-mile trail race. I had also gotten a bad rash on my legs and torso from poison oak. We visited my parents a few days later, and they insisted I see their doctor. I went in without a list of questions, got an X-ray that showed no break, began visiting with him about my parents, and forgot to ask about the poison oak. I paid dearly for that omission all

850 miles of the way home from Sacramento, as I dabbed completely ineffective calamine lotion all over my body while Karen drove.

Can I Get It Up (and Will It Stay Up)?

Every guy who undergoes treatment for prostate cancer, whether by way of surgery or radiation, worries about the recovery of sexual functioning. Prior to the availability of the nerve-sparing procedure, erectile failure was the routine outcome of prostate surgery. One friend said the surgeon told him something to the effect that, "First I'll save your life. Next I'll try to preserve continence, and after that, we'll worry about erections." The brother of another friend told her that he'd reverse the order of concern for incontinence and erectile dysfunction. Different people, different priorities. And of course, even with the nerve-sparing procedure, you may still lose the ability to get or maintain erections. One man I spoke with suggested, "In the weeks before your surgery, get your ashes hauled as often as your wife will allow, just in case."

Walsh notes that some doctors have men take Viagra® every night for the first year after surgery. He gave up this practice after not seeing much effect, limiting the drug to times when intercourse was planned. Dr. Golden told me to take the drug daily for a couple of weeks, even in the weeks before I would be cleared to have intercourse. Walsh does say that increasing blood flow in the penis helps encourage the return of the ability to have erections.

Your urologist and the relevant books will tell you that the ability to have erections will likely not happen all at once, but will improve as time passes after surgery. Sometimes this improvement does not show up for as much as a year. Of course, there are exceptions.

Some never recover function regardless of the use of the nerve-sparing procedure, and some do so surprisingly quickly.

Imagine a scene from a hopeful story. One man with whom I visited developed prostate cancer at 48 years of age and had surgery performed by Patrick Walsh himself. Imagine, if you will, this fellow lying in bed, a light cover over him in summertime, six days post-op. Streaming out from his penis is the plastic tube from the catheter in his bladder connected to the large bag pinned to the side of his bed. His wife walks by, partially clad, and he throws off the sheet and cries out, "Hey, look at this." The horny little rascal displays a full erection, catheter and all. His wife shakes her head and walks off chuckling; then they both are engulfed in a wave of sniggering giggles.

That's the end of the story, at least as far as I heard, though I wouldn't put it past him to have considered attempting some sort of anatomically unlikely action with his awakened little (or not so little) friend.

I know that I join tens of thousands of men and their partners in being grateful to Dr. Walsh for inventing the nerve-sparing procedure. Four years post-surgery, I am still able to get erections. Most of the time I do take the minimal 25 mg dose of Viagra, though sometimes things have been fine without it. I think that this is a very satisfactory outcome. (If you do go the Viagra® route, you can save money by having the medication dispensed in the 100 mg size and cutting it with a pill cutter if you are using a smaller dose.) I later thanked Dr. Golden and, indirectly, Dr. Walsh in the following poem.

ODE TO THE SURGEON

For twenty years
"anatomic" surgery
has removed prostates
while sparing the
tiny nerves that allow
You-Know-Who
to "be all he can be"
in the army of Amor
(though often with a
helping hand from
Big Pharma.)
Men worry about
post-surgical sex life and
while it's odd not to be
firing live ammunition,
Catholics can afford
to be dysrhythmic
and paternity suits
are no longer a worry.

About the quality of
his sexual experience
one nerve-spared fellow
wrote that while the
"whole orchestra didn't play,"
he could at least "hear the trumpets."
I consider myself lucky that
only the piccolo section
and a tuba or two
sometimes seem to get lost
on their way to the concert hall.

February 18, 2009[7]
Dedicated to Robert Golden, M.D.

---

[7] Previously published in the 2009 edition of *Blood and Thunder: Musings on the Art of Medicine.*

If problems with erections are not solved by pharmaceuticals, there is the vacuum pump. Briefly, you place a device over your penis which creates a vacuum and pulls blood into the erectile tissues. You place a rubber ring around the base of your penis to keep the blood from flowing out until after you are through enjoying yourself with your erection. There are also penile injections and penile implants that make erections possible. Some men will never be willing to try these methods, but others will find that they can have a satisfying time with them.

Whatever sort of medical help you seek, communication with your partner is valuable. It's likely that such communication was a contributing factor in a recent study of face-to-face and Internet-based couples counseling following prostatectomy or radiation therapy. The counseling led to significant improvements in a variety of measures of sexual function and sexual satisfaction (Schover et al., 2011).

If absolutely nothing works to allow you to have adequate erections, it is important to realize that as we age, the ability to get erections decreases anyway. While not having that ability is certainly a significant loss, and I am the last one who would diminish the importance of that loss, it is also true that you still have touching and other ways to give and receive pleasure that do not require erections. Finally, if you never recover the ability to achieve or maintain erections, or even if you can, for that matter, remember the lyrics from "This Is All I Ask," sung by Burl Ives, in which the old man asks "beautiful girls" to "walk a little slower when you walk by me."

Yes, if you still have your eyesight, girl-watching can remain fine recreation. Not that a sophisticated, high-minded intellectual such as myself would spend any time thinking or writing about such frivolous things as women's fashion, their style of locomotion, or their anatomy.

FETISH BY THE SEA

His lamentations (albeit unvoiced)
rang out along the promenade
as they paraded past:
slacks and pants,
trousers and toreadors,
jeans and capris.

Then she walked by,
not overly young,
not overly thin,
not overly pretty,
but in a dress,
by God,
in a dress.

Charleston, Oregon
February 15, 2009

And from Italy:

DIVINE WALKING
(though not upon water)

smoky latin siren
launches
haughty prow from
springbok limbs atop
fiery green stilettos;
skimpy silken skirt
flaunts
jaunty rhythm of
eye-bending strides—
I gape

Bologna Treno Platform #3
September 24, 2010

They say it's important to latch onto important memories and never let them go. Since I might have gotten smacked by Karen if she had caught me blatantly photographing this marvel of ambulation, I later spent a great deal of time writing and revising "Divine Walking" in order to capture, in the least number of words, my lone religious experience on our trip to Italy. Once again, it is hard to beat Italy for girl-watching. And then there is always nutrition for the fantasies.

MENTAL SNACK

olive-toned cleavage
Tuscany-based;
small, firm or bouncy
to suit every taste;
for those who are taller
strategically placed;
wickedly wanton or
naively chaste,
eye-candy refreshment
with no chance to taste.

Venice, Italy
September 26, 2010

Before we leave the subject of erections, I want to note that soon after Arnold Kegel devised his exercises for incontinence, they were also being used to help women who had difficulty reaching orgasm. In his informative and sometimes hilarious book, *Male Sexuality*, Bernie Zilbergeld (1992) also recommended these exercises for enhancing the experience of orgasm for men.

After a prostatectomy, you obviously no longer have a prostate (and probably not seminal vesicles, either) to contract, and such contractions have previously contributed to your experience of orgasm. Men report that even if things go well with regard to getting and maintaining erections after a prostatectomy, the sexual experience is altered, that their orgasms are lacking something after surgery. (Remember the poem, "Ode to the Surgeon?") Keeping your PC muscle toned may be one way to maximize the number and variety of instruments that show up on stage when you most desire to hear their music.

Regarding erections, in an early draft I wrote, "I haven't run across a correct anatomical name for the nerves in question, and you couldn't find them in classic anatomy texts, since Patrick Walsh didn't discover them until 1987. It does seem like they deserve a moniker with more pizazz than 'the nerves that control erections,' so I'm thinking of referring to them as 'Chip' and 'Dale,' after the mischievous cartoon chipmunks. The names would benefit from a play on words regarding those Chippendale strippers, who look like they have a pair of wool hunting socks or a two-and-a-half pound cutthroat trout stuffed down their tights. Also, the penis, with a mind of its own (remember the time at the blackboard in eighth grade when you couldn't turn around after finishing the math problem), certainly has a mischievous nature."

It's a bit disappointing to tell you that upon further research, I have found that the nerves in question are called "cavernosa nerves," which seems fitting, since two of the columns of spongy tissue in the penis that become engorged with blood to produce an erection are the "corpora cavernosa." I still like Chip and Dale, though— and everyone needs a nickname, right?

One thing is for sure. Let them remove your prostate, and you'll never take erections for granted again. Or as Jack Nicholson told Morgan Freeman in the popular movie *The Bucket List*, when you get old there are three things to remember:

1. Never trust a fart.
2. Never pass up a bathroom.
3. Never waste a hard-on.

I recently read the following comment posted in response to an online article about Viagra®. Obviously inspired by the above-mentioned movie, this person's humor may match Jack's wisdom: "If you're over forty, never trust a fart and never waste a hard-on. If you're under twenty, never waste a fart, and never trust a hard-on!"

As long as I am on this topic, I should tell you that while thinking about erections one day—hey, you need to think about a thing if you want to make sure you don't waste it, right?—I came up with the following:

BORROWED TIME

A British survey says
we most regret the
sex we did not have
when we were younger.

Life intrudes.

Sex,
like all of life,
is lived on borrowed time;
last long enough and
it will wax and wane,
and for the unlucky,
disappear.

If they yank your prostate,
yet crucial nerves remain,
sex can still be fine,
but if the threat of
salvage radiation

thrusts borrowed time
to the front of the mind,
you'll shield love's hours
from intruding life
and hope for more
waxing and less waning.

March 12, 2009

5

FOLLOW UP

Earlier, I described how my friend Bert, who had undergone a prostatectomy, had emphasized the importance of negative margins. Remember that a negative surgical margin (or simply, a negative margin) means that there is space between the last cancer cell observed and the edge of the tissue that was removed. Conversely, a positive margin means that the cancer cells run right up to the edge of the tissue that was removed, suggesting that there are additional cancer cells left behind after surgery. Unfortunately, as noted in the SURGERY chapter, I had a positive margin, and the cancer cells had also penetrated the capsule of the prostate. Even so, Dr. Golden had told me that the odds were 90 percent that my PSA would never go above zero.

I recall being apprehensive when I went to see him after having my first post-surgical blood draw to check my PSA. The draw had been a week or so earlier than the books recommended, but he assured me that it wasn't a problem. He asked how I was doing, how my continence was, and noted that the incision was healing nicely. Then he told me that my PSA was 0.37. His continued reassurance that I shouldn't worry was of little, if any, help this time. He said we'd re-check it in a couple of weeks. I spent a more anxious time before the next blood draw. My fears were confirmed when Dr. Golden called me on my cell phone to inform me of a 0.41 reading just as Bill and I were walking out the door of his house to run repeated all-out efforts up a steep four-tenths of a mile hill near his house.

I know that 0.41 sounds like a miniscule amount of PSA. Remember, though, that with the prostate removed, any PSA suggests the possible presence of cancer cells remaining in the body. Everything I had read had indicated that the limitations of the test indicated any value less than 0.02 was considered to be zero. A result of 0.41 was worrisome.

Dr. Golden also said that the above-zero result could be due to "free PSA." Free PSA is a variety of the enzyme that floats freely in the blood, unattached to other proteins, as is "bound PSA." Free PSA is not associated with cancer. It arises almost entirely from tissue that causes the non-malignant disorder called benign prostatic hypertrophy (BPH). He asked me to schedule a special lab test that could separate this "good" PSA from bound PSA, which is associated with cancer.

I hung up and gave Bill the news. We ran silently up the road toward our hill. Halfway there, I stopped and mumbled, "I can't do this. Go on without me." I jogged back toward his house. I wanted to stop crying before I called Karen. Just as I reached my truck, Bill ran up beside me. With tears in his eyes, he said, "I didn't want you to drive while you were upset. I was afraid you'd get hurt." We stood for a few moments. I said, "What the hell. Might as well go run." The leaden legs and burning in the chest from the hill repeats at least distracted me for a while. In fact, I ran my fastest repeats of the year that day.

It was soon after this that I changed my goals for running the Bloomsday 12 Km Run in early May. I had thought that, given my surgery, I would just jog the course rather than run my usual balls-to-the-wall, retch-at-the-finish effort. I had ramped up the intensity of my training for a couple of weeks, trying to improve my performance as quickly as possible while avoiding injury.

Karen and I were scheduled to pet-sit for Steven and Sue at their home south of Seattle for two of the last three weeks before the race. Every other day, we went to the Bonneville Power Company's power-line trail in Federal Way so Karen could walk Hershey while I ran. I mapped out a series of repeats of the trail that approximated the Bloomsday course and ran them at maximum effort every third day. It made for a good distraction, and I had about as good of a race as I could expect given the training, finishing under an hour.

My next PSA check on May 20, 2008, came back with a 0.20. Dr. Golden ordered a special radioactive test, called the ProstaScint® scan, that had been approved by the FDA in 1996 for, among other things, restaging patients whose PSA levels had risen following their prostatectomy. This scan is used to check to see if cancer cells have spread to other locations in the body. My scan turned out to be negative, which was reassuring.

On the other hand, despite the fact that one review article stated that, "ProstaScint® was found to be the single best predictor of positive lymph nodes in a study population at high risk for nodal metastasis" (Kipper, 2003), its use is somewhat controversial. The cost was about $2700. My insurance company refused to pay, labeling it "experimental/investigational," despite letters from Dr. Golden disputing this, letters from me containing a summary of supporting research, and an appeal in which I spoke with a panel by phone. I'll skip the details, but in the end, the State Insurance Commissioner's office told me that despite the fact that Medicare, Medicaid, Kaiser Plan affiliates, and many Blue Cross/Blue Shield carriers around the country covered this service, the insurance company could do whatever they wanted to do. Anyone for a single-payer, national health plan that takes the profit motive out of such arbitrary denials and spends a much smaller proportion of money available on processing claims, lottery-like CEO salaries, and other overhead? Wait, wait, wait. I was 64 years old when I had my prostatectomy. Now I'm 68, so I've already got one of those; it's called Medicare, and I'm glad to have it.

Past Reactions to Blood Draws

It's November 6, 2009. This morning I drove to Cancer Care Northwest to have blood drawn for a PSA test before meeting with Dr. Lee four days later. It's been six months since my last test. I took a copy of my order for my cholesterol test along. Might as well avoid an extra needle stick experience and save Medicare the cost of an extra blood draw. The phlebotomist joked with me that I didn't avoid anything, since she had to use my right arm after the vein in my left arm rolled over. I told her about being famous among family and friends for my reaction to the blood draw for the Wasserman test, when Karen and I eloped to Coeur d'Alene, ID, in 1964.

I was about ready to return to school at the College of San Mateo after a Christmas visit to Spokane, and Karen and I were tired of the long-distance romance after a year and a half. She had stayed in Spokane to finish high school when I went on to college. We decided to elope. We discovered that I was too young to get married in the state of Washington without my parents' permission. Talk about sexist. I was twenty, Karen eighteen. She could get married in Washington without permission. I suppose the theory was that women matured faster than men. My parents would gladly have given permission, but they were in San Mateo, and we wanted to get married right away, so that I could make it back to the Bay Area by Monday morning for my registration appointment for the spring semester.

Early Saturday morning, we picked up my wedding ring, bought Karen a new suit, and got my best friend, Mike, and his girlfriend, Marilee, to drive us across the border into Idaho. At the Presbyterian Church, Reverend Winkle told us we needed to go the courthouse and obtain a license, but before that, we had to have a Wasserman test to rule out syphilis.

At the lab, Karen went first. Then it was my turn. As soon as they extracted the needle from my arm, everything began to go black. The technician caught me on the way down. I suppose the stress of figuring out the eloping process may have contributed to my nearly passing out.

My reaction didn't fit with my past history with blood draws. When I was a young child, I had monthly blood draws to measure the sedimentation rate, a measure of inflammation important in the assessment of rheumatic fever. During my first bout with the disease, my sister also had it. An iconic family story has been that I always was the one to go first, readily sticking out my scrawny arm without evident distress. I still get a little light-headed when blood is drawn. I always remember to be sitting down for the process now.

Oh, yeah. We did get married, and by driving a spanking-new rental Chevrolet straight through, we made it to the Bay Area in time for me to register for school Monday morning. We never went back to visit Reverend Winkle. When I saw that he died a couple of decades ago, I regretted not visiting him to tell him that those two kids had made it together, and happily so, for over 40 years. There's another lesson for us all. When you think about contacting someone or doing something for someone, don't hesitate. You never know when one or the other of you will be gone.

In June and August of 2008, my PSA levels had dropped to 0.10. Once again, overall, I had good success in terms of putting the chance of cancer recurrence out of my mind. Denial is often a destructive coping strategy.

However, I figure that when you get the result you want from your PSA re-check, there isn't much that worrying about what might happen at the next one can do for you. I decided to focus on the things I could control, such as getting good sleep, drinking my red wine and pomegranate juice, taking Vitamin D, eating soy-based meat substitutes, fish, lots of fruits and vegetables, and no red meat. (More on dietary choices later.) Other than that, I tried to ignore the likelihood that there were still some malignant cells trying to fight their way into dominance. Big surprise—I wrote the poem on the next page for the occasion.

DENIAL

With six months
to wait till my next PSA
I recalled I could
frame things
in one helpful way:

Denial is
dangerous,
deadly and
dumb
when used to avoid
things that need
to be done,
yet a very fine answer
to worry's distaste
after you finish
what you know
must be faced.

February 25, 2009[8]

---

[8] Previously published in the 2011 edition of *Blood and Thunder: Musings on the Art of Medicine.*

The calendar continued to loom large in my head, though. In the two or three weeks prior to each PSA check, my thoughts returned unbidden to the idea of a PSA rise and further treatment, namely external-beam radiation therapy. Though I know it seems rather melodramatic, the necessity to have recurrent PSA tests does evoke an image of the Sword of Damocles hanging over my head. Or, to put it poetically:

THE NUMBERS OF MAN[9]

Earlier our notable numbers
were batting average, salary and GPA.
In middle age they shift to
cholesterol, years till retirement and PSA.
Don't be fooled, the last stands for
Periodic Stimulation of Anxiety.

February 28, 2009

That's okay. I did a good job of keeping those worries at bay during most of the interval.

Time's A'Wastin'

As a psychologist, I always questioned the validity of paper-and-pencil research that asked people what they would do in different circumstances. We know that people often do not behave as they think they would when confronted with something. Nevertheless, some researchers have based their entire careers on publishing studies based on this strategy. I remember at my follow-up, after approximately four and one-half months, my PSA had decreased from 0.20 to 0.10. Before learning the

---

[9] An earlier version of this poem was published in an article about my therapeutic writing and prostate cancer written by Virginia de Leon for *The Spokesman Review.*

results, I was thinking that I should have a huge party to celebrate if the number came back low. I also anticipated experiencing enormous elation.

The PSA check came and went. The reading had even decreased to "less than 0.10" by late October, which Dr. Lee said was equivalent to zero given the sensitivity of the test. My reaction was relief rather than euphoria, and I didn't get around to throwing a party. The pattern repeated in the spring at my first follow-up for the longer six-month interval.

Last Friday, I had my blood drawn as noted above. I'll meet with the radiation oncologist tomorrow to learn the outcome. Over the last ten days or so, I have again noticed big party fantasies occurring and found myself anticipating euphoria if I get good news. I haven't let the idea of bad news spend much time residing in my brain. It will be interesting to observe my reaction after tomorrow's appointment.

Despite any worries or concerns, my job—and the job of anyone else with a chronic or life-threatening disease—is to keep on living, getting the most I can out of each day I continue to breathe.

Dan Fitzgerald died last week. He was one of those larger-than-life, one-of-a-kind guys. He did two stints of coaching the men's basketball team at Gonzaga University, setting the foundation for the spectacular success this small school's teams would later achieve. I had been an Instructor in Psychology there from 1969 to 1971 and returned as an Assistant Professor of Psychology in 1978, the same year that Dan returned for his second time as the Bulldogs' coach.

In 1979, I got to know Dan when I taught a course called The Psychology of Running, which counted as credit in both the psychology and physical education departments. That year, he invited me to be the university's cross country coach. Unfortunately, because I was running a private practice in addition to my teaching, I could not find the time. I appreciated the offer, as that job would have been tremendous fun. In addition, if I would have stayed on at the university, I would now possess good seats to watch what has become a national powerhouse basketball team. I sure as heck can't afford to buy seats now. Karen and I later worked closely with Dan for a number of years when he was running the silk screening company that printed the 50,000+ finisher shirts for the Lilac Bloomsday 12 Km Run that Karen directed for 13 years.

There are many in our community who think that Dan was treated poorly by the men in the tight white collars. When I first arrived at the school, I expected that these "men of God" would treat faculty members with fairness and compassion. Indeed, I was treated in a reasonable manner both times that I was a member of the Gonzaga faculty there. Unfortunately, I found out that I was naïve, and that the Jesuits were human, just like the rest of us. Sometimes their treatment of their employees was less than perfect.

According to an account by Bud Withers (2002) of *The Seattle Times*, Dan was left hanging for months, unsupported by the university over a slush fund that he used to support his team during some very lean years. After a thorough investigation, the NCAA called for probation, but in Withers' words, the organization did not levy "serious sanctions." And even with his death, the university's tribute to Dan seemed half-hearted to many. Withers quotes Fitzgerald regarding the university leaving him in limbo for a protracted time, then offering to give him a job in some other area. "If they had fired me 30 seconds after they found out, I'd have some respect for them. But to go through what I went through, the expense of it . . . and then to offer me a job back. I said, 'There's not enough stamps for me to lick.'" (p. 47)

I remain a rabid GU basketball fan. We never miss a game; heck, we even attended two games in southern California when we were vacationing there a few years ago. Still, I wish that the situation with Dan would have been handled differently. Dan was a dynamo, a gregarious, exuberant storyteller who lived life to the fullest. He did much to help others in the community.

Dan's death highlighted for me the way in which my medical concerns seemed to have moved me toward a water-treading approach to my own life. I would never claim to have possessed the charisma or the limitless vigor of Fitz, as he was more often known, but the health issues have had a noticeable effect on how completely I have been living my life.

Today I was thinking that this is a great example of the conditioned suppression definition of emotion I discussed earlier. The emotion is shown by the disruption in the ongoing behavior. My inner, personal experience of this phenomenon is probably best captured by words we use, such as depression, anxiety, or anger, but it is fascinating to note how well the conditioned suppression model described earlier fits here as a completely objective, observable measure of the effect of these events on me. Here is my tribute to Dan in verse.

SQUANDERED DAYS

A revered basketball coach
died last week; an
energetic,
optimistic,
enthusiastic, yes,
bombastic
heart
told its final tale
in a local eatery.

Dan Fitzgerald
devoured life in
MASSIVE BITES.

Cancer diagnosis,
obsessions
about treatment,
recovery
from surgery,
waiting
for lab results
and delayed
heart operations
reduced me to
nibbling
around the edges
of my last two years.

RIP, Fitz

January 24, 2009[10]

    Again, it's bad enough to waste your time when you have lots of time left. It's much worse to fritter away days when it's likely that you are going to run out of days earlier than you had planned. So why allow history, habit, and impulse to steer your ship? Take charge, even if that means sometimes allowing yourself to not be in charge of, for example, emotion, which rather than being suppressed, can be experienced and expressed.

    Cancer Care Northwest is a modern, high-quality treatment center. I found the people there to be dedicated professionals. It has a relaxing, though fake, aquarium in the waiting room, plus free coffee, tea, and hard candy. And I hate walking in its door. Let me repeat: I hate

---

[10] Previously published in Spring 2009 edition of *SpokeWrite.*

walking in its door. This morning, I was recalling the second time I drove into the parking lot. Karen and I had been there several months earlier for our consultation with Dr. Lee when I was still in the decision-making mode. I remember being anxious, but not overly upset. We were there together to gather information.

The second time I met with Dr. Lee was to consult about external-beam radiation therapy, since my post-surgical PSA was still at 0.31. As I started to get out of the car, I had a smothering sensation. It wasn't that I had difficulty breathing. It was more like a weight was pressing down on me all over, a sinking black hole in the center of my being with a dark cloud circling overhead.

As I have tried to put into words what was going on inside me, I realized that part of it was that at that moment, I felt more alone than I have at any other time in my life. Each time I have gone in for a PSA or a consult at Cancer Care Northwest since, I have experienced this feeling, though to a much lesser degree.

I think that part of my reaction to the clinic is related to denial—a refusal to believe that I belong in such a place. Most of the people look very ill. Many are in wheelchairs, some with oxygen. Some seem halfway through Death's door. Hell, I feel great. I can still run reasonably long distances, hike, and hunt and work hard. Yeah, I get tired more quickly, go slower and need longer to recover, but that seems to be a normal part of the aging process. But come on, these poor bastards have cancer!

Oh yeah—so do I.

I had a similar experience at the first appointment with Dr. Goldberg in 1992. Running in the annual Turkey Trot five-mile race with my son-in-law, Dwain, I had a heavy feeling in my legs and had to stop for a few minutes. After several other similar occurrences when I was running hard over the next couple of months, I finally went to the doctor. It was clear from a stress EKG that I had tachycardia of some kind. I had been referred to Dr. Goldberg to determine whether it involved the atrium (which would have been more of a nuisance, possibly requiring me at most to take blood thinners to prevent a stroke from the blood swirling around because of the uncoordinated action of the heart) or the ventricle (which would have been much more serious, ventricular tachycardia having been the cause of death of two great basketball players: Hank Gathers of Loyola Marymount, and Reggie Lewis of the Boston Celtics).

Dr. Goldberg began examining me, occasionally commenting to the medical student who was following him. At one point, I think I said out loud something such as, "I don't belong here. I'm an ultrarunner. I run 50 and 100 mile races in the mountains." I'll bet that later in the day, he used me as a prime example of denial to his young charge.

At this radiation consult, I found myself sticking my head in a magazine while in the waiting room at Cancer Care Northwest. The woman accompanying the man sitting across from me was quite loud, almost histrionic. Her phlegm-ridden, octave-too-low croak was a walking neon sign that said: "I am a smoker." The thought crossed my mind that it's that sort of person who should have cancer, not me, and maybe not the man she accompanied. Sounds familiar—same old theme as that in "Whiny Lifestyle Lament" back in the DECISION chapter, doesn't it?

I immediately reminded myself (here comes another example of countering irrational self-talk) not to be so judgmental. Whatever her lifestyle habits, she was there helping someone she cared about. That says a lot about her in my book. Besides, as you probably concluded from the poem "Poop Occurs" in the SURGERY chapter, I do believe that the universe is merely random in the sense of lacking an overall guiding purpose toward which it moves, though not in the sense of lacking lawful relationships between its parts.

True, our behavior can make us more or less likely to have bad things happen to us. Nevertheless, neither disease, misfortune, suffering, nor death is doled out based on whether people deserve such a fate or not. On my way out the door, another young woman was helping a tall, stooped old man from a van into a wheelchair. He sported a brilliant maroon beret. The color was a severe contrast to his pasty, near-translucent skin. I had an image of him as a tanned, strapping young man glowing from work under a summer sun.

I stopped, leaned over to make eye contact, and told him that I loved his beret. It was fun to get a smile from him. It must not be that easy to smile while strapped to an oxygen tank. The woman said the beret was a something-or-other that I couldn't quite make out, but it was the kind Mel Gibson wore. I managed to smile and leave without presenting my views of Mel Gibson and his radical Catholicism. Hey, good for me. Maybe by reminding myself to engage people, if I have to come down here, I will find it less oppressive.

6

BIOCHEMICAL FAILURE

SALVAGE RADIATION

I really hoped that I would not have to include this chapter, but here I am, and I'm doing it. I suppose I could have avoided doing so if I had spent more time writing and completed this manuscript earlier, but then I would have omitted a big part of my story. On the other hand, who wants to have the word "failure" attached to their condition? And don't most people wish to avoid the necessity of being "salvaged"?

Then again, how do you know when it is time to finish any sort of memoir? I suppose the only way to tell the entire story would be to keep writing until a couple of seconds before your last gasping breath and have your family publish it posthumously, but then you'd miss out on the thrill of seeing your work in print, as well as the "big bucks."

But writing to the very end seems to be what the irascible, irreverent comedian George Carlin did. George died in 2008, only a few days after being named the eleventh recipient of the Kennedy Center Mark Twain Prize for American Humor. His autobiography, *Last Words*, was still in progress, to be finished by co-author Tony Hendra after George was gone. Speaking of "Last Words," George wanted the following on his tombstone: "Gee, he was here a moment ago . . . ."

I can't resist including a poem I wrote in 2009 on the same topic:

LAST WORDS

It's too much to ask to come up with a closing line
to equal John Adams's "Jefferson still survives,"
even if that was not quite true
on that pre-internet/pre-Twitter
50th anniversary of the Declaration of Independence
when Adams couldn't have known
that Jefferson had died earlier in the day.

It would be tacky to plagiarize Walter Lance with,
"Buh-duh, buh-duh, buh-duh, That's All Folks!"
and "Yo Jesus, wassup?" doesn't seem quite right, either.

I wonder how many leave this realm
calling out "Momma," an echo
of the word with which they began?

My Dad's "Oh, oh, my back, my back" when his
abdominal aortic aneurism exploded
was certainly no match for the
raunchy one-liners from the rest of his life.

So I'd like to excel in this area of Last Words,
but rehearsing seems unseemly.
Would it be better to trust to spontaneity
when the time arrives?
No, after all this talk, failing to prepare a final speech
would be like trying not to think of a pink elephant,
so I'll work at it.

Unfortunately, "Hello Darkness, my old friend"
has already been taken, though in different context.
I'll probably make do with,
"Oh Fuck, I always knew this was going to happen."

After a year or so had passed since my surgery, I began to wonder if maybe my pre-PSA anxiety and dread would diminish as time went by. After all, I was a psychologist, an expert on anxiety management—wasn't I? On the other hand, I had written a poem a year after my surgery that suggested that it might not turn out that way. Here's how that came about.

The article in *The Spokesman Review* about my poetry project for prostate cancer has just been published, and Karen and I are staying in our trailer at Sunset Bay Campground on the Oregon Coast. There is no cell phone coverage in the campground, but I stick my cell in my pocket, as is my habit ever since I had my private practice, when I needed to be available for crisis calls. We finish breakfast and hike up through the forest overlooking the raging Pacific.

As I follow Karen up the soft, soggy trail, everything is a muted green, and the rain is dribbling down my neck inside my coat. Hershey is scrambling through the dense underbrush in search of the nearest rodent. It's hard to be in a bad mood when that big brown doofus is so joyfully living in the moment.

I'm thinking that I am rarely happier than I am walking with Karen and Hershey at the ocean, when I am startled by my phone. We have rounded a high bluff and must have caught a better angle to a tower in nearby Coos Bay. Gary Higley, a high school friend, is calling from Spokane. He has just read the newspaper article. He relates his own prostate cancer story, including his prostatectomy seven years earlier. I suggest that he write some poetry about his experience. "Hey, Steve, I got a "D" in English from Mrs. Praetorius. I can't write."

Karen is getting irritated that I have to stand in the rain in this one particular part of the trail to maintain reception. To keep us moving, I end the call without my usual cajoling to convince him that he can, indeed, write a poem. I return to the trailer and write the following verse in honor of Gary, our friendship, and our new connection as prostate cancer survivors.

HOME FREE?

A year after my own surgery
I asked a high school friend
about his prostatectomy.

"It's been seven years.
I was one of the lucky ones:
totally encapsulated
and all my PSAs have been zero."

"Congratulations; you're home free!"

"You're never home free.
It can always come back.

I think about it every day.
If I have a pain,
say in my hip,
I wonder.

You're never home free."

February 12, 2009

At my PSA check in the spring of 2010, six months after my previous test and about 27 since my prostatectomy, my PSA had risen from 0.10 to 0.20. At that point, I wrote the following: "It's approaching two and one-half years since my prostatectomy. Because my PSA levels have never gone to zero, I've been going through the repeated wait and see anxiety-producing cycles every six months. This recent slight increase, which may or may not be significant, has decreased my testing interval to four months. In addition, as noted above, over the last year I have dealt with the same sequence of Diagnosis, Decision, Surgery, and Recovery issues with regard to heart disease. I suppose any memoir could continue on until the person wrote the last sentence right before his heart stopped on his death day. I'm all for closure and would like to see this published, so I am going to wrap it up."

Obviously, I have yet to "wrap things up," and, despite some amount of repetition, I kept the preceding material to allow you to get a sense of the ongoing nature of dealing with prostate cancer, especially in cases when you do not have Gary's good fortune of having repeated zero PSA values.

Decision Time Again

Five months later, my PSA score had increased to 0.30. The only possible good thing to say about these data is that they seemed to motivate me to spend more time working on this book. On the other hand, it feels like *déjà vu* since I found myself once again researching articles on the Internet concerning when and if to have radiation. If you have biochemical failure after a prostatectomy, i.e., your PSA has risen beyond a certain amount or increased on three successive measures, one option is to have radiation, which is then called "salvage" radiation.

Once again, it does not appear that there is a black-and-white, all-or-nothing, right-or wrong decision to be made about the treatment or its timing. I found articles stating that the outcomes for salvage radiation depend on a variety of variables, and one consistently mentioned is having the radiation before the PSA rises too high.

You will recall the discussion in the DECISION chapter about the controversy surrounding the use of PSA as an initial screening device for prostate cancer. At this point we are talking about something quite different. Here, the focus is on the value of the PSA *after* the person has been diagnosed with cancer and had his prostate removed. Some researchers stated the importance of having this salvage treatment while the PSA is still below 1.0. A number of others place the range between 0.20 and 0.40. The one comparison I have yet to find is between people who have the salvage radiation and those who have no treatment at all.

All the studies I have found only relate outcomes to these variables, such as positive versus negative surgical margin, capsular penetration, pre-radiation PSA, and the like. Dr. Lee said that my three successive rises would lead any radiation oncologist in the country to suggest that it was time for external-beam radiation therapy.

I had met with his nurse practitioner for the main part of the appointment. When she went to get Dr. Lee, I noticed on the computer an order to schedule me for a bone scan and a pelvic and abdominal CT scan to make sure no metastasis had occurred. For some reason, when I saw the words "Rule out MET disease," it was the first time that I really, really, really, really, reeeally believed, way deep down that I had cancer. Weird? I know, but that was the sense I had. As usual, I have used writing to help me deal with my disease. You knew it—here's a poem.

MAN OVERBOARD

When a third post-surgical
rise in PSA earns me
an invitation for

an eight-week ride
in the radiation Tilt-A-Whirl,
I know I should
ignore the extra
chills and thrills with
lovely names like
strictures, fecal incontinence
and rectal bleeding;
should be grateful
that it is possible while
sun-burning my rectum
(Dr. Lee's phrase)
to ravage malignant
adenocarcinoma
with ionizing rays
akin to those
that gave Madam Curie
her Nobel (before killing her),
but it's hard to hear
"salvage radiation" without
feeling like a
mud-mired,
barnacle-crusted
shipwreck.

October 22, 2010

After reading a number of articles without finding the
information that would help me with decision-making
(and after my friend Bill said, "You probably aren't going
to find that information because the science probably
hasn't been done"), I emailed Dr. Lee asking for

references to any articles with the control groups I wanted to see. I also emailed Rob Golden, and he called me with his views, which went something like this:

"Steve, there's not a lot of detail regarding just watching after a prostatectomy. The research is anecdotal. If it were me, here is what I would do. I'd have the PSA re-measured every three months. If it doubles in three months, then seriously consider radiation therapy. A three-month doubling time represents a significant prostate cancer recurrence. If it is just creeping up, though, say doubling every 12 to 18 months, it can take a long time, like 10 to 15 years, before you have trouble spreading to the bones or other places. There is significant morbidity with radiation and with hormone therapy. Of course, the longer you wait, there is an increased chance of spread of the disease. At these levels, living with the uncertainty is a better option than radiation. But also, remember, you can't make a wrong decision here. Call me any time you want to chat."

External-beam radiation therapy involves the kinds of risks listed in the "Man Overboard" poem, and hormone therapy is commonly accompanied by such changes as decreased energy, softening of bones, hot flashes, loss of libido, and cardiac problems. A further side effect of hormone therapy is illustrated by a poem from 2008 that was based on a discussion I had with Bill Greene.

HORMONAL IRONY

As Bill and I discuss my concerns
that I'll need hormone therapy,
complete with hot flashes,
if salvage radiation after
my prostatectomy fails,
he says, "It's like you pay the price
for being a male,

then get the penalties
of a female, too."

"Yeah, and with the
gynecomastia[11] and loss of libido,
the hormones will plop
my very own set of boobs
onto my chest,
but I'll lose interest
in playing with them."

June 14, 2008

At this same visit, Dr. Lee had invited me to participate in a research study comparing three combinations of external-beam radiation therapy and androgen deprivation, or hormone therapy, each of which had been previously determined to be successful. Deep down, I knew from the moment I took the paper describing the research study that I wouldn't agree to participate. Sorry, Science. I love you, but . . .

True, I have no doubt that the scientific method is one of mankind's greatest inventions. When the beta-blocker Tenormin® failed to do an adequate job of controlling my ventricular tachycardia in 1992, I didn't hesitate to try sotalol, a new beta-blocker thought to have more specific anti-arrhythmic properties, even though it was an investigational medication. I was a part of an experiment in which I had a two-day hospital stay to be carefully monitored, since a few people had died on sotalol. That worked out well. The drug, later branded as Betapace®, controlled my arrhythmia and allowed me to run safely, while decreasing my speed by maybe 10-15 percent. I ran more than 20 ultramarathons, including 17

---

[11] Gynecomastia (or gynecomasty): abnormal enlargement of the breast in a male.

Le Grizz 50 Milers, on sotalol. I have been on this drug for 18 years. This is a long enough period for the drug to run out of its patent, so that I have been able to buy the generic brand very inexpensively for over ten years.

With this prostate cancer study, however, I could not see any advantage in participating. If my cancer was very advanced and there were no established successful treatment regimens available, I very well might join a clinical trial of a promising new treatment. Here, however, I would be randomly assigned to one of three regimens that had been successfully used. A head-to-head comparison with the gold standard of random assignment was aimed at the question of whether they differed in usefulness.

I suppose it came down to that old question of control—having control or the *semblance* of having control. I did not want to add hormone therapy at this time, if I didn't need to. Hormone therapy was an adjunct to radiation therapy in two of the three options. Thus, I had a two-thirds chance of landing in a group that involved hormone therapy. I wasn't willing to take my chances with regard to random assignment in order to make a contribution to gods of Science. I suppose this attitude has some selfishness to it. I can live with that.

My bone scan was clean. We looked at it on the computer screen. It was the first time I had looked at my whole skeleton. Weird. More than weird. For whatever reason, I got quite anxious when looking at it. The CT scan of my abdomen and pelvis showed a variety of metal surgical clips from my prostatectomy, as well as small areas that were most likely to be cysts in my liver and kidneys.

It also showed a couple of tiny (5 mm or less) areas along the sides of my prostate bed in the lymph node areas. These were just noted, and Dr. Lee said there was no evidence to suggest that they were cancerous. We just didn't know. I was a bit alarmed. The specter of occult metastases seemed palpable. However, he said, "This is a good scan. This is the kind we like to see."

As we discussed treatment options, Dr. Lee said something such as, "There is controversy about (I've lost this part), but there is no controversy about whether or not to start radiation therapy in your case." The second important thing that he said was, "I will support whatever decision you make regarding treatment, including getting no treatment." I appreciated that.

I told him that I thought I wanted to wait three months and re-check my PSA. We decided to check my PSA that day, as well. It had been one month exactly since the test that showed the rise to 0.30. He also ordered a complete metabolic panel and testosterone level. I had never had a testosterone measurement (other than indirectly, through my competitive style and my incessant horniness for my wife, I suppose), and that might be a useful baseline. I realized when reading the research proposal that these blood tests and the rectal exam he did that day were the measures that would be done at the beginning of the research study, so I suppose he was getting prepared in case I decided to join the study.

One morning, it dawned on me that it would be useful for me to once again prevail upon my second cousin, Bryan Maxwell, and his wife, Jen Liu, who were still at Stanford. In her third year of residency, Jen was certainly up-to-date on the most cutting edge research.

I emailed them an update of my case and requested her input. Despite an undoubtedly crushing schedule, she took the time for a thoughtful reply. Regarding the option of waiting for another PSA check, she noted that there were cases in which a small amount of benign prostatic tissue was left behind in surgery, but she was also clear that if I waited for another PSA check and got a further increase, I should begin external-beam radiation at that time.

After discussing the pros and cons of immediate external-beam radiation therapy, she summarized her position. "Okay, hopefully that has not muddled the situation more. I tend to agree with your urologist in that I don't believe that there's a definitive answer. But I do think there's a 'right' answer in terms of your own feelings about cancer and treatment side effects, and what you consider to be acceptable for your lifestyle."

I had difficulty sleeping for a couple of weeks while I stewed about whether to begin radiation therapy at that time. I finally emailed Dr. Lee and told him that I was not going to be a participant in the research study and was going to schedule a PSA check in mid-January, two months after my latest check. I immediately began sleeping well each night. Whether nutrition is a critical factor or not, I decided to tweak my diet a bit so that, if nothing else, I could feel that I had done everything I could to counter my cancer before becoming involved in radiation therapy. I'll summarize the diet stuff below.

Karen and I had finally given in to our desire to buy a small motor home to replace our trailer. We drove it to the Seattle area and spent a wonderful Christmas with the kids and grandkids at Steven and Sue's new house, up in the woods outside of Fall City. We then went to Portland and watched McKenzie play several basketball games. Afterward, we spent eight nights on the wild Oregon Coast. We were thinking that since I might end up spending two months in radiation therapy, we should get in a trip to the beach while we could. We lucked out with relatively easy winter driving by traveling between snow storms.

I'm noted for being frugal (some would say cheap), so some people were quite surprised that we spent what for us was a pretty good chunk of money on a motor home. Earlier with regard to my heart surgery, I wrote how the realization that you may have much less time left than expected reminds you how important family, friends, and experiences are as compared to material possessions. Now I'm telling you that I purchased the most expensive item I ever have, other than a house.

Maybe the following comment from my psychologist friend, Chuck Lund, has influenced me: "I'd rather run out of money before I run out of time than to run out of time before I run out of money." On the other hand, I don't think it is a complete rationalization to view the motor home as a means for garnering a greater number of experiences.

I had the blood draw for my PSA on Monday, January 10th, and saw Dr. Lee the next day. Over the weekend, I was reminded of my poem that stated that PSA really should stand for Periodic Stimulation of Anxiety. When the medical assistant came in before I saw Dr. Lee, she said my PSA was "really good—0.20." That meant that it had dropped. I was ecstatic. I was close to tears and almost kissed her. I was hoping for no change, and any decrease was phenomenal from my point of view. When Dr. Lee came in, he asked me how I was. I said, "Really great now, with a 0.20 PSA."

Dr. Lee said that my PSA was 0.30, not 0.20. Fascinating how everything is relative, how we anchor our judgments. For example, consider last year when Joe had heard that his Christmas bonus was going to be $500. Imagine his reaction when he opened the magic envelope and found four one hundred dollar bills. Now imagine how he would have felt about receiving $400, if he had been led to believe that his bonus was going to be $50.

In a similar fashion, if I had not been previously told 0.20, I would have been quite pleased with 0.30. Now I was disappointed. On further reflection, though, I was able to shift my perspective back to being reasonably satisfied that there had been no progression. Dr. Lee indicated I could still begin external-beam radiation therapy at any point, if I chose to do so. I was certain that I wanted to wait and re-check in three months. We'd pet- and house-sit for Steven and Sue the first part of April, and then return to have another PSA check after that.

So at this stage of my writing, that's how things stand regarding treatment plans. To stay with the program of gathering more experiences, we also spent an additional two weeks on the Oregon Coast before the April test. In fact, in yet another aside, I'll tell you that I am writing these words at Sunset Bay Campground on the 50th anniversary of our first date. It's just a few days after the earthquake killed over 10,000 people in Japan, and the tsunami here didn't cause us any problems, so it's seems pretty petty to be whining about any of my health problems. That's what you call perspective.

A few weeks later, I was shuffling through some papers and ran across the lab report Dr. Lee had given me. I started to file it away, and then in my typical compulsive fashion, I glanced over the list of prior test results that had been penciled in below the current value. It appeared as though one was missing.

I noted also that this sheet contained a testosterone reading, which I did not think had been ordered at the last visit. Dr. Lee had mentioned that my testosterone level was in the mid-range of normal, and when I asked him why it was tested again since it had been measured in November 2010, he said something about the importance of knowing if it was too low if a person was undergoing hormone therapy. While I still didn't understand why the test was done, this was a time when I did not persistently speak up until I understood.

Now, as I looked at the lab report, I noticed that the date read "11/10/2010." I was sure he had referred to the wrong lab report in January. I called Karen in and asked her to look at it just to make certain. Yep, this was the November, not the January, report. It's easy to see how someone could see "11/10/2010" and not notice that it was supposed to be "01/10/2011." I immediately called Cancer Care Northwest and asked to speak with Dr. Lee's nurse. When she called me back, she confirmed that the January test result was indeed 0.20, just as the medical assistant had stated.

Any frustration that I had about office paper-work mistakes or doctor error was washed away by my relief. Again, we are talking about very small values, and the amount of change was tiny, but the testing is supposedly more and more precise, and it was at least in the direction that showed a reversal of the ominous trend. Obviously, I am postponing external-beam radiation therapy again, at least until the planned PSA test after three months.

Consider another example of how dramatically our perspective can change. I remember times when I was certain that if I was told I could not run and compete in ultramarathons and other races, that I would have been devastated. Now here I am, finding it difficult to run more than a few times a week, three to five miles at a time at a *very slow* pace.

The other day, I realized how much more focused I have become on just being able to live a longer life, and to do so with the least amount of distress from my cancer or the treatment undertaken to fight it, than I am about any sort of athletic aspirations, abilities, or shortcomings. That may not seem surprising to people who have never made a substantial commitment of time and energy competing or striving for an athletic or fitness goal, but it represents an unexpected outcome to me.

I found A. J. Jacob's *The Year of Living Biblically* to be relevant to the issue of living with a life-threatening disease. As in my poem, "Three Little Words," when Jacobs focuses, albeit in an extreme, obsessive way, on all he can be grateful for, he sees it as a reminder to himself to "Pay attention, Pal. Savor this moment." (2008, p. 269)

You don't need to focus on being thankful that the elevator arrived quickly, didn't crash into the basement, rose to your fifth-floor destination without stopping at other floors, and on and on and on, as A. J. did. But I know that since my diagnosis, I make a stronger effort to look around and experience fully whatever it is that I have before me right here, right now. I also am better at not taking for granted the relationships and conveniences that I have in my life. That's a shift in perspective that will pay off as we deal with our disease. Here's a poem I wrote while waiting for the April PSA.

DEADLY GUEST

How strange to live with a killer;
how odd to share space with
a part of you bent on
destroying the whole of you,
mindless
suicide terrorist replicator
primed to slay the body
in which it dwells,
to cut off its nose
(and all else)
to spite itself.

When the tests claim that
some cancer was
left behind after surgery,

some tiny specks
of renegade cells
dividing,
re-dividing,
re-re-re-re-re-re-re-dividing
unduly fast
(or maybe not-so-fast,
that's the Big Question),
it's hard to escape the image
of these wild little bastards
as they dodge killer T-cells,
as they slip-slide their silent way
out from the cozy prostate bed,
as they ascend along
the aorta highway;
it's a trick to elude
the echo of these rogues
as they ricochet
off to their favorite haunt,
your spine,
for their final assault.

At moments it seems
you might reach inside
to pluck them out

with your fingertips,
with micro-tweezers,
with a teeny golden spoon,
or maybe an onco-magnet,
but there is no magic,
and when your
derelict vessel can
no longer be salvaged
through radiation,
what remains are
girlie chemicals eager
to brittle your bones,
to fill you with flames that breed

empathy for your tormented wife,
and yes,
to sprout you some
splendid ya-yas all your own.

When all's been done
that will be done,
that can be done,
you're left with prayer
if that is your wont, but
I don't and I won't,
even should options
dwindle to merciless misery
or narcotic haze.

How strange to thrive in this
living-with-a-killer world--
though mindful of the evil
that grows within,
to defy terror that
feeds on what may await;
to look not back nor
toward your yet-to-be,
but at this moment, this day,
for that's all there is,
and all there ever was--

to LIVE.

March 27, 2011[12]

It's been about three weeks since I wrote "The Deadly Guest." I had my blood drawn a couple of days ago. Today, Dr. Lee reported that my PSA was 0.30. Here is a table that tracks my PSA, beginning five weeks after surgery.

---

[12] Previously published in the 2011 issue of *Blood and Thunder: Musings in the Art of Medicine.*

1/29/08	surgery
03/05/08	0.37
04/10/08	0.41
04/20/08 (approx.)	0.31 ("free PSA=zero)
05/20/08	0.20
06/17/08	0.10
08/15/08	0.10
10/20/08	Less than 0.10
05/01/09	0.10
11/16/09	0.10
05/11/10	0.20
10/13/10	0.30
11/10/10	0.30
01/10/11	0.20
05/??/11	0.30
11/03/11	0.36

I was a bit disappointed that the level hadn't stayed at 0.20 or dropped to a lower value. Again, however, the absolute values here are very small. Dr. Lee said that it might actually be no different from that of last time. It could have been 0.24 last time and 0.25 this time, with the value reported differently based on rounding up or down. He also remarked that the PSA just seemed to be sitting around near that low level and suggested I might let my family physician follow it at this point. If it went higher, I could then call Dr. Lee. He said that whatever cancer is in there is growing very slowly, that a six-month interval made sense, and that he wasn't worried about it at this time.

I assume that when the upward trend that had been occurring over the previous year leveled off, he became much more comfortable with my postponing any further treatment. So I am going to be grateful that my "Deadly Guest" is behaving himself for now and work at forgetting about him and his pals until it's time for a re-test in the fall. In the meantime, of course, I will continue the same regimen I have been following. Who knows, maybe I can reach the goal Dad always talked about when he said he wanted to die at 95 years of age, being shot by a jealous husband. You can see where I get my raunchy humor.

Obviously, I inserted the 11/03/11 data point in the table on the previously page some time after writing the last paragraph. As you can see, my PSA had made another tiny jump at that time. I continue to postpone any further treatment, with a re-check scheduled in March 2012.

7

CAUSES AND PREVENTION

This chapter moves us back a step from the phases of diagnosis, decision-making, and surgery to the issues of cause and prevention. The most desirable path is to avoid the disease in the first place. So what are the biggest risk factors? Two of the most significant are things over which we have no control: race and age. It is well established, for instance, that men whose modern ancestors came from Africa have the highest incidence of prostate cancer. This effect is strong enough that they are advised to begin PSA screening earlier than are Caucasians. At the other extreme are Asian men, who have the lowest incidence of this disease of any racial group.

There are clear indications that some men have a strong genetic tendency, unrelated to race, to develop prostate cancer. However, this genetic influence only affects a minority of the men who develop prostate cancer.

Age is also strongly related to the incidence of prostate cancer. The older you become, the more likely you are to develop the disease. Walsh and Worthington (2007) state that in the two decades between 40 and 60, an American man has a 2 percent chance of developing prostate cancer, while in the next two decades, the incidence rises to 14 percent.

There are a variety of other factors that are implicated in prostate cancer that can be controlled. While the research data may not be as clear-cut as are those with race and age, the evidence of the importance of these elements seems to be growing. For example, where you live makes a difference. Northern latitudes tend to have a higher incidence. It is suggested that this is related to a lower exposure to sunlight, and thus, less Vitamin D. This idea is compatible with the fact that men with dark-skinned bodies, which produce less Vitamin D in response to sunlight, have an increased incidence of the disease.

What about other lifestyle variables related to prostate cancer? One of the most telling criticisms of the lifestyle of Americans and of our health care system is that too often the focus is on fixing things *after* they go wrong. Many people make scant effort to live their lives in ways that decrease the chances of a variety of diseases. Instead, they merely go to the doctor and expect to be fixed with a pill or procedure. For example, cigarette smoking, not wearing seatbelts, unprotected promiscuous sex, abuse of alcohol and other drugs, keeping loaded guns where children can access them in the home, obesity and sedentary habits, and a variety of dietary choices are strongly implicated as harmful to our physical well-being.

The crisis of our rapidly rising health care costs could be at least in part ameliorated by an upsurge in the number of people who acted proactively to prevent chronic illnesses. Not only would the economic situation improve, but people would see a dramatic enhancement in their quality of life.

This section is related to prevention of prostate cancer. However, a similar approach of personal responsibility for education, for creating a collaborative relationship with your doctor, and for appropriate lifestyle change is important with regard to most other maladies as well. I encourage you to become actively involved in doing whatever you can to improve your health, and especially to combat prostate cancer. As an example, if you need any further motivation to quit smoking, I give you the recent study (Kenfield et al. 2011) showing a correlation between smoking at the time of prostate cancer diagnosis and an increased death rate from prostate cancer.

Earlier I mentioned that I was following some specific dietary practices to try to slow the spread of any cancer cells that might be remaining after my prostatectomy. I have not found these changes to be drastic or onerous. We haven't eaten significant amounts of beef or pork for decades, for example. Don't get me wrong. Down deep in my heart of hearts, I believe that the ideal diet would be made up of chocolate chip cookies, peanut M&M's®, ice cream, Doritos®, and beer. Maybe if I am told at some point that I have six months to live, I'll go in that direction. I might even smoke one of them there maryjuanna cigarettes at that time to see what that experience is like.

In the meantime, I'll follow the suggestions that seem to be the healthiest. Mostly, this involves food, since the choice of what we eat on a daily basis does seem to show promise in regard to prostate cancer risk. Meat, especially red meat, dairy products, and partially hydrogenated oils found in packaged foods seem to have the most evidence of harmful consequences. In particular, the intake of animal fat from red meat and dairy products increases the chances of developing advanced prostate cancer, and of dying from the disease.

Soy, green tea, fruits and vegetables (especially blueberries, tomatoes cooked in olive oil, and cruciferous vegetables such as broccoli, cabbage and cauliflower), red wine, turmeric, and Vitamin D appear to be nutritional items most likely to play a role in prevention.

I found a recent newspaper article fascinating. The author was suggesting that people cut down on their meat eating. He suggested starting by having meat at only one meal per day, then gradually shifting to having some days with no meat, until meat was on the table only three times per week. The implication was that people could learn to do this, but it would be very difficult. Wow, what a difference that is from the way we normally eat. Despite my healthy lifestyle, I still got prostate cancer, and it has been difficult for me to avoid searching for some way in which I might have screwed up. The earlier poem, "Assigning Blame," helped me with this somewhat obsessive issue.

A year and a half after my surgery, my Ph.D. dissertation chairman, Grayson Osborne, commented in an email, "Just keep drinking that pomegranate juice." I had no idea what he was talking about, so I checked with him, and he said there was some recent research about pomegranate juice and prostate cancer. Pomegranate juice is apparently very high in antioxidants, just the sort of thing to fight the free radicals that contribute to cancer.

One study was done in vitro (i.e., in glass, in a Petri dish) in which pomegranate juice added to prostate cancer cells slowed down the growth of the malignant cells and sped up apoptosis (cell suicide). In one encouraging example reporting over five years of data, men with prostate cancer who drank pomegranate juice after experiencing a post-surgical rise in PSA had a four-fold increase in the time that it took for their PSA to double. Before beginning the pomegranate regimen, the average PSA doubling time was 15 months. At the end of the study, it had increased to 58 months. In addition, the PSA doubling time of men who continued to follow the program after the end of the study

206 | R. Steven Heaps Ph.D.

increased to 69 months as compared to 51 months for the rest of the men (Dreher 2008).

Patrick Walsh's writing showed me how animal fats did their damage. Apparently, prostate cancer cells contain an enzyme that thrives on the fatty acids found in dairy products and red meat. If you have prostate cancer and eat a lot of meat and dairy products, your cancer cells receive nine times more energy from these foods than do normal cells. The cancer cells also produce hydrogen peroxide, which damages DNA. You then get more mutations of cells and a worsening of your cancer (Walsh and Worthington 2007, p.46).

Picture this. You have a monster from a science fiction story that you must defeat. You sit down to dinner with this mortal threat. You have always liked a certain dish, and so you serve it. Not only have you enjoyed the dish, but it has also given you strength in the past. Unfortunately, you discover too late that your special food provides this vile brute with many times as much power as it does to you.

Oxidative damage and inflammation are two major foes against which our body's defensive arsenal must be turned. These factors are important with regard to cancer. It wasn't until I read Walsh's book that I also learned about a wonderful enzyme called glutathione-S-transferase-π, or GST-π, for those of us whose tongues get twisted by lengthy chemical names. Remember that it is damage to normal cells by the oxidative process from free radicals that feeds cancerous growth.

Walsh notes that a colleague in oncology at Johns Hopkins discovered the role of the GST-π enzyme in neutralizing the effects of free radicals. The GST-π is not found in prostate cancer tissues, highlighting the value of this protective enzyme. Cruciferous vegetables such as broccoli, cabbage, cauliflower, kale and (I know, yuck)

Brussels sprouts all contain sulforaphane, which increases GST-π. So eat your broccoli and cauliflower.

Even though it's way too late for me to *prevent* prostate cancer, some of the same sorts of choices that show promise regarding prevention also appear likely to retard the growth of cancer cells when you have experienced biochemical failure after surgery or radiation. I recently saw reference to a study by Dean Ornish, the physician best known for his work with lifestyle factors and cardiovascular disease.

Many years ago, Ornish presented the first evidence backing the success of diet, stress management and exercise, not only for slowing down the progression of atherosclerosis, but for actually decreasing the amount of plaque clogging arteries, which has since been verified by PET scanning methodology.

A few years ago, he published an article (Ornish et al. 2005) evaluating the effect of similar factors on prostate cancer. A group of men with prostate cancer consumed a low-fat vegan diet for one year. They also followed a regimen of aerobic exercise and stress-management techniques. Their PSA levels actually decreased by 4 percent, while those of a control group increased by 6 percent.

While these are small changes in absolute terms, the shift in the direction of the trajectory of the PSA as a result of the lifestyle regimen seems very promising. In addition, six of the men in the control group, but none in the experimental group, required further treatment of their cancer during the study period.

Paul Lange, a renowned urologist at the University of Washington, speaks to my two central points—attitude and a sense of control. After performing thousands of prostatectomies, Lange underwent the same surgery, an experience which he says increased his empathy for his patients. Referring to the work of Ornish, Lange commented, "Even if scientific evidence is still meager, complementary medicine approaches have strong appeal in practicing the medical art, since they give the patient an active role in his care and promote an attitude of optimism and hope." (Rob Stein, *The Washington Post*, August 11, 2005)

During this period of postponing external-beam radiation therapy while carefully monitoring PSA levels (again referred to as "post-surgical watchful waiting"), Karen and I have paid even more attention to the kind of food that we eat. (Of course, she doesn't have to worry about prostate cancer, but the food choices that seem best for prostate cancer are very similar to diets that appear to be the best for cardiac health and health in general.) I am lucky to have a wife who is not only a talented and creative cook, but who has always shared my interest in healthy eating. Karen has faithfully crafted meals that are delicious and in line with what appears to be the most likely diet to retard prostate cancer. I do help with meals, though more often I only do the cleanup.

I have continued to avoid eating meat, other than a small serving of chicken (or turkey during the holidays) once or twice a month. I also will eat any pheasants, quail, partridge or grouse that Hershey and I are able to bring home, but the reduced bird populations and my marksmanship are adequate protection from my consuming large amounts of these delicacies. I have added a 1000 mg capsule of pomegranate and pomegranate seed extract marketed as POMx® to my diet and have done a better job of increasing eating fruits and vegetables. I have reduced the amount of dairy products, especially cheese, and am phasing in soy milk, though we have drunk skim milk for the last four decades.

I have increased my vitamin D dosage to 2000 mg and drink one or more cups of green tea daily. I am adding turmeric to various dishes. For lunch, I more often than not eat miso soup or sauté stewed tomatoes/tomato sauce in olive oil with black beans or rice, cauliflower, broccoli, and carrots or other vegetables. I continue drinking one or two glasses of red wine most nights.

I have friends who cannot imagine avoiding meat, but I don't feel deprived eating this way. I am also careful to indulge myself to a small degree. I will eat a handful or two of barbequed potato chips or nachos before dinner every once in a while, but don't eat many more than that. I eat a small amount of dark chocolate frequently, and a few cookies a few times per week. I think I am covering nearly all the bases concerning the prevention and countering of prostate cancer.

Unwittingly, I have also been following one additional regimen that appears to fight prostate cancer. Farwell et al. (2011) reported that that taking cholesterol-reducing medications called statins reduces the risk of prostate cancer, especially in cases classified as high grade. I have taken statins for over a decade.

The dietary suggestions related to prostate continue to appear, with the latest research pointing to coffee (Wilson et al. 2011). Researchers found that men drinking six or more cups of coffee, whether caffeinated or not, developed the more lethal varieties of prostate cancer at a lower rate than did those who did not drink coffee. I doubt that I will increase my coffee consumption to that extent, but it certainly suggests that a cup or two per day isn't going to cause prostate cancer problems.

These practices may turn out in the end to have greater or lesser importance than we now can predict. Regardless of all this, and this may be beginning to sound repetitious, I hope you have picked up on the idea that making these various dietary choices represents one more way in which a person can have a sense of having control over something, even if the amount of actual control turns out to be illusory.

There is an increasing amount of evidence appearing regarding the effect of diet on our health and illness, including the incidence of cancer. However, as with many aspects of medicine, much of the evidence about diet and prostate cancer, especially regarding cancer that remains active after surgery or radiation, is regarded as tentative, if not speculative.

For example, a study appeared on line at www.cancernetwork.com on April 27, 2011, reporting completely counter-intuitive results concerning the relationship between omega-3 oils found in fish and prostate cancer. These oils have previously been touted for possible help with prostate cancer. In this study involving 3,400 men, those with the highest levels of omega-3s had a much greater risk of aggressive prostate cancer, but not of low-grade prostate cancer, than did those with the lowest levels. These data are in marked contrast to the studies reported by Walsh and Worthington in their discussion of causes of prostate cancer that showed a clear benefit to eating moderate to high amounts of fish. This was especially true with cancer that had metastasized.

The Selenium and Vitamin E Cancer Prevention Trial (SELECT) is the name of a prostate cancer study involving over 35,000 men, which has been ongoing since 2001 (Klein et al. 2011). This experiment includes the gold standards of research, random assignment and blind, placebo controls. For years, I remember hearing about selenium and prostate cancer prevention. This SELECT research did not show a benefit of taking selenium. Somewhat surprisingly, men taking 400 units of Vitamin E had a significantly increased incidence of prostate cancer. I had been taking that amount of Vitamin E on a somewhat irregular basis. These findings convinced me to not take any Vitamin E supplements in the future.

I realize that such changing outcomes make many people throw up their hands in frustration and eat anything they want. I'm certain you, like I, have heard people whose self-talk in such situations is *See, none of these things work. It's all unclear, so I am going to go ahead and eat and drink and live any damn way I want.* I certainly can appreciate that point of view. Rather than lamenting the frequent reports of studies that show ambiguous or even contradictory data, my response in this case has been to moderate my intake of omega-3 fish oil tablets, taking them now and then rather than daily.

I also have thought about another issue that comes out of the psychology lab. In the absence of a clear-cut, rock-solid relationship between time of survival after recurrent prostate cancer and diet, there remains the possibility that following such a diet may be what psychologists call "superstitious behavior."

Superstitious behavior is a set of actions that continue because they were accidentally followed by a positive reinforcer (or by the removal of a negative reinforcer), even though there is no connection, no dependent relationship between the behavior and the reinforcer. The behavior doesn't produce the reinforcer; it doesn't have to occur for the reinforcer to follow. The behavior continues, though, because of this accidental or "adventitious" reinforcement.

As noted above, this phenomenon is seen in the animal behavior laboratory, and is commonly demonstrated by such human silliness as wearing a lucky bowling shirt, stepping over mother's-back-breaking sidewalk cracks, and rain dances. On the other hand, since there is at least some evidence for the value of the sort of diet plan I am following, and no evidence that it is harmful, I will continue on this course.

Rereading Walsh's prostate cancer book recently, I came across the following information about prevention that I must have read three years ago. I find it astounding that I did not remember this monumentally valuable material. Walsh notes that scientists have suggested that frequent ejaculations make the gland less vulnerable to substances that promote inflammation and thus, cancer. He further noted that Harvard researchers reported that men reporting more frequent ejaculations had only two-thirds the risk of prostate cancer of that of men who reported less frequent ejaculations.

Several months after I read this information, we were watching the movie *Days of Darkness*, filmed in Quebec. Jean Le Marc is a burned-out government bureaucrat who tries to spice up his life with outlandish fantasies. His wife has cuckolded him and then run off with her boss. Jean is hiding from the tobacco police, sneaking a smoke with two coworkers, a black male and a lesbian. The black male warns Jean that he will "catch cancer" because he doesn't have a woman, based on the theory that males are created to need to ejaculate once every three days. When the lesbian asks him for evidence, he claims that Japanese and Koreans have the most sex, and also the least prostate cancer.

My guess is that the screenwriters thought they were writing an outrageous joke, and that they would be astounded to learn their vignette has scientific support. This unlikely coincidence made the joke especially funny for us.

Of course, both the movie character's claim and the research cited by Walsh only show correlation. I took enough statistics classes to know that correlation does not necessarily mean causation. For example, both outcomes could be related to an unrecognized third variable. In this case, for example, maybe increased smiling is related to a lowered incidence of prostate cancer. But, I'm not saying that you have to tell your wife about the possible limitations of this correlational research. In fact, if I would have had access to these data throughout the last 48 years, I might have used them as part of a seduction strategy with Karen. Can't you just see it? I'd burst through the door after a trip to the library and exclaim, "Hey, Honey! Guess what I just read about preventing prostate cancer?" Of course, those who know my wife could predict that she would retort with her trademark, "Yeah, in your dreams."

8

THE FUTURE

The future for men with prostate cancer is more hopeful than it ever has been. I marvel at the improvements in my lifetime. In his landmark book, Patrick Walsh credits early detection via the rectal exam and PSA testing with saving thousands of lives. A few decades ago, those diagnosed generally were not diagnosed until they were older, and men often died after only a few years. Outcomes have improved to the point that Walsh states, "*Now, most men are diagnosed with localized prostate cancer that is curable. It is possible today to prevent a man from dying a painful death of prostate cancer fifteen or twenty years in the future.*" (Walsh and Worthington 2007, p. 218-219)

After a prostatectomy in those earlier times, a man was routinely expected to be incontinent and have problems with erections. Not so today. Further advances, both in surgical techniques and in employment of newer imaging procedures for both diagnosis and radiological treatment, continue to improve these outcomes. A variety of personalized pharmacological approaches that interfere with cancer progression have been developed, and clinical trials are ongoing for even more of these methods, which bring great promise for the treatment of advanced metastatic disease. For a recent summary, read Rush and Hussain (2011).

For me, the future is also bright. I will continue to get my PSA evaluated on the schedule recommended by my oncologist. I will continue to follow the lifestyle and dietary habits that I think have the best chance to strengthen my immune system. Who knows? I may be able to avoid radiation or other further treatments. If my PSA does rise significantly, I will have further treatments available that can at least delay the progression of the disease. In the meantime, to use the title of Edmund Fantino's book about his prostate cancer, I will focus on "behaving well."

As mentioned before, Fantino learned that there was a great deal of variability in length of survival in different reports of men with his sort of aggressive cancer. True, the predicted overall average time of survival for him was short, but again, that was just an average, and an average says nothing about one individual case. He decided that given this unexplained difference between different men, there was a good chance that he was an outlier, or would be so if he followed the dietary and lifestyle program that was likely to enhance the function of his immune system. He decided to assume he would be around for five years.

One of the ideas that he put into practice in his own case was to divide the rest of his life into five-year blocks, and to set goals for one five-year block at a time. You can read his example in his useful book. On the other hand, this is my book, so I'll give you a tentative five-year goal list of my own.

1. Enrich my relationships with Karen, my kids and their spouses, with my grandkids, my siblings, and friends.

2. Complete this book, submit, rewrite, and resubmit it until it is published.

3. Use our Frequent Flyer Miles for our long-planned trip to Europe. (This one was completed in September 2010 with a great time in Italy; France is next.)

4. Visit Alaska.

5. Visit the Southwest of the USA.

6. Go pheasant hunting in North or South Dakota or Iowa.

7. Take a motor-home trip across the USA.

8. Continue to raise money and award scholarships for the Joseph Heslin Foundation in memory of a beloved teacher and coach.

9. Read one serious book about science, philosophy/religion, literature, politics or history each month.

10. Maintain fitness

11. Write poems, short stories, essays.

12 Revise my "Emotional Wills" annually.

11. Become involved in a new volunteer activity.

14. Sell or give away possessions rarely used.

15. Finish the inside of the cabin.

Note that the second item on the list refers to finishing this book. This project can be seen as an attempt to derive meaning from my disease.

Joe Agostino has been my friend since Mrs. Boberg's fourth grade class. In the spring of 2011, I learned that he was going to have a prostatectomy, and I communicated with him about my experience. During high school, Joe and another classmate of mine, John Beam, became somewhat notorious for starting two radio stations, one in each of their basements. Of course, they did so without the blessing of the FCC. Joe got caught and received a cease-and-desist order, along with the threat of a huge fine and something like 15 years in prison. "Jockey Joe" was the disc jockey for our high school sock hops and went on to a career in TV and radio, specializing in producing commercials and making documentary recordings.

During his recovery, Joe decided that he did not get enough information about what to expect from prostate surgery and recovery. Rather than merely whine about this oversight, Joe is producing a video, for which he interviewed me and a half-dozen other men who had had prostatectomies, aiming for a guys-talking-to-guys approach to discussing things that aren't easy to talk about, such as fear and helplessness, sexual functioning, and incontinence. He also is filming a surgery for the DVD, which should come out in 2012.

He plans to market this documentary to physicians, asking them to distribute it to their patients. Hats off to Joe for combining his expertise in producing documentaries into a product that will aid others. His project also provided an opportunity for us to renew our friendship after nearly five decades.

I think *The Rancid Walnut* and Joe's DVD are akin to the work of the lady who founded Mothers Against Drunk Drivers (MADD) in response to her daughter having been killed by an intoxicated driver. Meaning is found in these lemonade-from-lemons endeavors.

Some people say that having cancer, or becoming paralyzed, or some other such traumatic experience is the best thing that ever happened to them, because it changed their view of life, made them appreciate life more, or led them to God. I'm reminded of Voltaire's Pangloss. Remember him—an important character in the novel *Candide* (1959).

True to his name, for Pangloss, everything that came along, no matter how horrific, was for the best in this, "the best of all possible worlds." Toward the end of the book, he is confronted about this view. "Tell me, my dear

Pangloss," said Candide, "when you were hanged, dissected, cruelly beaten and forced to row in a galley, did you still think that everything was for the best in this world?" His answer: "I still hold my original opinions." (p. 114)

Well, I certainly don't adhere to such a world view, nor do I believe that "everything happens for a reason." And as I said before, the notion of a personal God who involves Himself or Herself in the daily life of humans remains unlikely to me. Sometimes, you are just randomly dumped on by the universe, as described in the poem, "Poop Occurs."

So overall, I think that getting cancer basically sucks. Since we're all terminal anyway, and we spend a lot of time avoiding thinking about the reality of our own fragility and mortality, a diagnosis of something such as cancer or heart disease can be a wake-up call, reminding us to live more in the present, rather than always looking forward to tomorrow or next year or looking back with regret, resentment, or remorse. The disease can also put many things about which we worry or become angry into perspective. For me, cancer also got me to place extra focus on that which is most important to me—namely my family and friends, to appreciate them and tell them so.

The vast majority of the writing and advice about prostate cancer concerns early detection and the choice of the appropriate treatment for each person. Earlier, I addressed the usefulness of early detection as well as the differences of opinion concerning screening and biopsies. Suffice it to say that regardless of the concerns about unnecessary biopsies due to early screening, I wish that I had been more diligent in following up when my PSA rose the first time. (I started to write, "I would give my left nut . . ." but I thought that might over-stretch the reader's pun tolerance.) If I had followed up sooner, my cancer might have been less advanced, and I might have had consistently zero PSA readings after surgery. If so, it is unlikely that I would have written the preceding chapter.

Also, if I had never had a PSA above zero after surgery, I doubt if I would have been focused enough on the issue to even begin a book such as this. I think my reaction might have been similar to what I think that of many of my friends in this position has been: pay little or no attention to the cancer, except right before the annual PSA test. I guess I can say that at least I got a book out of the way the disease progressed.

In the book *Authentic Happiness,* Seligman (2002) presents a great deal of evidence to show that people are really quite poor at predicting what will make them happy. For example, ask college students how they will feel if their team wins or loses Saturday's big football game. Now wait until a few days after the game, and ask them how they actually feel. Inevitably, they don't feel nearly as sad after a loss or nearly as happy after a win, as they had predicted.

Similar results appear when the predictions are made concerning more momentous life events, such as becoming paraplegic or every parent's worst nightmare, the death of one's child. Again, we may not be able to change a lot of important things, but we can have some say about how we cope with those things. The CBT methods for managing emotions and behavior described in this book are designed for just that purpose.

I have talked a number of times about the importance of taking control of things in your life. Even the illusion of control can be comforting. However, sooner or later, we all end up in a place in which we have little or no control of anything outside of ourselves. In the case of prostate cancer, you may have controlled everything that you can, for example, in terms of diet, compliance with medical regimens, exercise, and so on.

Yet sometimes the most important, or what seems to be the most important, thing cannot be controlled—what your cancer does. At that point, we are still left with the one thing we can control. We can, at least to some extent, choose to be happy. It would be an error to assume that this is as easy as just making a one-time choice. That is not what I mean. It is more about making the choice of setting out to choose our actions and the way we think to maximize our happiness, to create meaning in the rest of our lives. And that is what matters.

I urge you to read Victor Frankl's *Man's Search for Meaning* (1963). Frankl recounts his experiences in a concentration camp in Nazi Germany. If there is any other situation in which one has less control over events than being in such a place, I can't imagine what it could be. Frankl shows, though, that there were still choices to be made, and it was those choices which created meaning and helped him survive this horror. Though he founded the psychotherapy of Logotherapy from these experiences, he was basically doing cognitive-behavioral psychotherapy, although in a less systematic fashion.

Each day, no matter what the circumstances, I think it is our job to choose to engage in behaviors and manage the things we say to ourselves, in ways that create our own meaning and happiness. So, if I survive for the five years, my Mini-Bucket list will have provided a useful guide for living a life according to my values.

Hopefully, I will have completed the entire list in five years. After five years, I can make a new list which can include ongoing goals, such as numbers 1, 10 and 12 above, along with any goals not yet attained, and any new goals that strike my fancy. If I die in less than five years, I will at least have had a plan to motivate me to spend those years doing things that are important to me, rather than waiting, waffling, wandering, and worrying. With this approach, I don't see how I can't lose.

Regardless of the condition of your health or how long you think you are likely to live, I challenge you to go through this Five-Year Mini-Bucket List exercise. Get out your paper and pen now. Doing so will be especially useful if you feel yourself adrift, vaguely unsatisfied, or searching for meaning. Again, how can you lose? Of course, there is nothing sacred about the five-year interval. Choose some other time span, if you wish. Your list may bear no resemblance to mine. Who says it should? It's your list. Go for it.

Self-Control or Self-Management

How do you get yourself to stay on track, to make progress toward your goals? What do you need to do to maximize the quality of each and every day that you have left? And how do you decide what goals to work toward in the first place?

First of all, you do need to choose some goals you want to pursue. Otherwise, you join the legion of your fellow humans who drift along from day to day without a clear picture of where they are going. It is surprising how many people fail to take even this first step. I suppose a strategy of drifting along has its advantages, but I believe that people often come to it by default, rather than via a conscious decision. I believe we can lead more satisfying lives if we are deliberately following a plan pointed toward how we want to be and how we want our lives to unfold.

So, what gets in the way of our living full lives? Dysfunctional emotional reactions such as depression and anxiety certainly interfere, regardless of whether or not we have a major health problem with which to cope. With the Seven Cs, I have already presented proven CBT techniques for altering moods. Now I want to spend some time showing you in more detail how to add methods that will help you avoid drifting, and instead take specific steps to increase actions that you value, and limit those that are incompatible with your goals.

One of the key principles arising out of the work of B. F. Skinner in operant conditioning is the notion that behavior is a function of its consequences. The events that follow an action play a major role in determining whether that action is more likely or less likely to occur in the future. Consequences that increase the probability of behaviors that produce them are called positive reinforcers, and those that decrease that probability are designated negative reinforcers, or punishers.

Thus, the way in which our world is organized to provide these differing outcomes goes a long way toward explaining, predicting, and controlling how we will act in a given situation. Tell me what typically results from someone's action, and I can make a good guess about that individual's future behavior. Let me have control over what the consequences are, and I will have at least some degree of control over what the behavior will be later on.

One of the biggest problems for humans involves the question of self-control or self-management. In writing this book, I knew that a major theme I wished to address was the use of psychological methods to help men deal with prostate cancer. In *Behaving Well*, Fantino introduced men to self-control methods for living a full life in the face of life-threatening disease.

I had spent my entire career teaching self-control methods to students and psychotherapy patients. I had written handouts and papers and given workshops and presentations explaining these methods. Though I will cover some of the same ground that Fantino covered, I will do so in a somewhat different manner, describing several additional strategies and including more specific examples of self-control techniques, along with a stronger emphasis on the integration of the self-talk methods of CBT. After discussing the biological facts that make such strategies necessary, I will present several of these strategies.

Many of the things in the world that act as positive reinforcers to strengthen our behavior are attractive to us, because way, way back in our history, it was to our ancestors' evolutionary advantage to go after these same things. For example, consider the survival value of obtaining high-calorie, fat-laden, sugary food in a world in which obtaining a sufficient number of calories was a priority of the first order. Our nervous system evolved along with such a world so that the pleasure centers in our brain light up when we stick some of that stuff in our mouths. It's a darn good thing that was the case in primitive times, or we wouldn't be here.

In the modern world, this characteristic presents a problem, though, because we still have the same brain, susceptible to react in the same way to these substances in a world awash for many of us in cheap, fatty, and extremely unhealthy meals.

The need for self-control can be quickly summarized as follows. As a species, we are wired to be reinforced by the immediate changes that follow our actions. Thus, we are predisposed by the very structure of our brains to seek outcomes that provide immediate rewards, even though they may be small, rather than to delay our gratification in order to receive larger rewards at a later time.

Self-control is essential in many areas of our lives, in addition to that of nutrition. To use a modern example, the problem with credit cards is that they take advantage of a dangerous flaw built into the brain. This failing is rooted in our emotions, which tend to overvalue immediate gains (like a new pair of shoes) at the cost of future expenses (high interest rates on the credit card we used). How long does it take to receive enjoyment from the video game in front of you, rather than studying? How long does it take to experience the rewards of getting an A at the end of the semester instead? No contest, right.

Or, imagine you are standing at the big box store, gaping at the giant screen TV/home theater system. Just a quick swipe of your credit card, and soon you can be sitting in front of your very own cornucopia of entertainment. How can the near-immediate excitement of this marvelous set-up compete with a healthy IRA account that you won't access for decades? Impulsivity wins again.

Conversely, we gravitate toward activities that provide immediate rewards when negative consequences which accompany them, though sometimes catastrophic, are long delayed. Smoking cigarettes, lying, gambling, promiscuous sexual activity, and using narcotics fit here.

Another principle almost always included in any behavior-change program involves setting intermediate goals, so that a sequence of small steps of progress is strengthened as you move toward the ultimate goal. When I would ask my psychotherapy clients the question, "How do you eat an elephant?" they would often give me a look that suggested that we should switch chairs. They got it, though, as soon as I continued, "One bite at a time."

The Problem of "Will Power"—We often hear people describing people they admire with terms such as hard-working, efficient, or having a lot of "will power." They add, "I wish I had his will power," or "I can't get my work done (or stop smoking or exercise and so on) because I don't have enough will power." When people speak this way, they are viewing will power as a quality or trait, and that is a dead end. They mistakenly believe that you either have it or you don't. If you do, lucky you. If you don't, too bad.

I prefer the term "self-control" (or "self-management"). At least as early as the 1950s, psychologists were talking about self-control and ways to develop the skills that defined it.

My first introduction to the study of self-control came in 1966, when I read Skinner's classic *Science and Human Behavior* (1953). This book extrapolated to our daily lives the principles of conditioning which Skinner had been studying for years in the animal laboratory at Harvard. Written nearly sixty years ago, this book still stands as a model for what we can do as we move to demonstrate the relevance of these laws of learning to the real world.

Skinner discussed self-control in terms of a person doing some action (a *controlling* response) that changes the probability of some other action (the *controlled* response). I will provide several examples in a minute. In general terms, then, self-control involves arranging your environment in such a way that you end up performing the actions and experiencing the feelings that you desire. I will use the terms self-control and self-management interchangeably.

Richard Powers was one of my graduate school professors. We lived across the street from him and his wife, Elki, for three years while I pursued my Ph. D. at Utah State University. They have been dear friends to Karen and me for over 40 years. Richard required each of his Introductory Psychology students to complete a self-control project. Each student had to choose some behavior and conduct a program to observe, record, and change that behavior. In this way, they received hands-on, practical experience in applying to their own lives basic principles of behavior that were originally formulated in the animal laboratory.

226 | R. Steven Heaps Ph.D.

I followed Richard's example when I taught at the University of Manitoba and at Gonzaga University. My students successfully modified behaviors such as studying, swearing, cigarette smoking, being nice to others, exercising, and playing the piano. Before taking my course, many of these young people would have ascribed their prior failures at such behavior-change efforts to a lack of will power. At the end of my course, they thought differently.

Think about watching your brother-in-law, Ralph, lying on the sofa watching NASCAR rather than looking for a job or studying to make himself more employable. Or imagine offering your four-year-old the choice between either three M&Ms right now, or 33 of them tomorrow. Little Johnny will usually take the ones you are holding in your hand rather than wait. In each case, you might say that the person has little will power. They both are choosing an immediate, smaller reward over a larger reward for which they have to wait. And each of them loses out in the end (though you may be happy that Johnny didn't choose to wait a day and then pig out on eleven times as much candy).

<u>Making a Commitment Response</u>—What about birds? What if I tell you that I can teach a pigeon to exhibit the same behavior you are wishing to see in these humans in your life? I'll tell you how this form of self-control has been demonstrated in pigeons.

Among all the tedious research papers I read during graduate school, one of the exciting ones was published by Rachlin and Greene in 1972. They first described the unsurprising finding that if you give a pigeon a choice between a situation in which a peck on one key yields the immediate opportunity to eat grain for two seconds, and a situation where a peck on another key earns twice as much time to feed, but only after a four-second delay, the birds overwhelmingly choose the smaller, immediate reward. They look just as undisciplined as Little Johnny, or your sister's beloved lump. A lack of avian will power is costing these birds 50 percent of their potential food. No big surprise, you say. I agree.

Rachlin and Greene next rearranged the birds' world in a way that allowed them to develop self-control. They were provided with another choice, this one coming before they got the opportunity to choose between the smaller, immediate and larger, delayed rewards (SI-LD.) This new choice allowed them to go forward into the SI-LD choice situation as before, or to put themselves in a situation where they had no choice but the larger, delayed reward. The latter choice, restricting oneself in a way that one only has the option of waiting for the larger, delayed reward (showing will power, if you will) is called making a Commitment Response.

Karen and I would probably have been unable to retire if we had not for decades had mutual fund companies take money from our checking account automatically each month. If we'd had that money in our pockets every month, we would have been more likely to spend it. We make similar Commitment Responses whenever we make promises or sign contracts.

When the pigeons were given the opportunity to make a Commitment Response 16 seconds before they had the chance to put themselves in a situation where they were "unable to help themselves," they came to choose the more mature, better-in-the-long-run, self-controlled path by making the Commitment Response over 80 percent of the time. A variety of studies have replicated and expanded on this phenomenon. There you go. Birds can learn self-management.

If you have prostate cancer or some other serious disease, I suggest you use the methods of managing your emotions and behaviors I have outlined. And even if you are in perfect health, why not follow the same path? Every one of us is terminal, after all. This might be a good time to re-read "Three Little Words" in the DIAGNOSIS chapter. My message to you is to stop talking about not having this thing called will power, and get busy rearranging your world in ways that lead you to make choices that are in your long-run best interest. Use these methods as a way to move each item on your five-year plan from an idea to a series of progressive steps toward your goal. If a bird-brain can do it, so can you.

Of course, you are the one who will choose the particular behaviors you wish to include in your life. This is where the values by which you live come into play. I will relate an anecdote from sometime in the 1970s which illustrates how one could use this self-control strategy for a somewhat questionable goal. While there have been over three decades of controversy between the men about who played which role in this escapade, the basic facts of the behaviors that occurred have never been in question.

It's a nippy November day late in the upland bird hunting season along the Palouse River in southeastern Washington. Two young psychologists have been slogging along for hours without sighting a single bird. With each step, their boots break through the snow's crust with a raspy crunch. The low winter sun still has the power to take the edge off the sting on their rubied cheeks. As they round a bend in the river, they spy a dozen brilliantly bedecked roosters roaming an acre's worth of brush-covered island. Pheasant Heaven. The hunters begin salivating like Pavlov's dogs, but soon notice the ice that covers the width of the stream. The water underneath may be only a foot deep. It may be seven feet deep. There's no way to tell.

"Okay. Let's go get 'em."

"Yeah, let's. You first."

"Whaddaya mean, me first? Don't be such a weenie. That ice is okay."

"Sure it is, Wimp. Go ahead. I'm right behind you."

"Wasn't I the one that tested that rickety bridge up on Billy Goat Mountain last summer?"

"Are you kidding? I remember you whining like a little girl up there."

At this point, Psychologist #1, the skinny one with the big nose, recalls the Commitment Response technique and decides such a strategy is in order. He unloads his 12-gauge and lays it in the grass.

"Let's take some time and think this over. Lemme see your gun."

"What?"

"Lemme see your gun, just for a minute. My stock seems too short. While we wait, I want to see if your gun fits my shoulder better."

Psychologist #2 hands over his weapon.

"Be careful. It's still loaded. Just because I accidentally shot your dog last year doesn't mean I want to get shot."

Before #2 can protest, #1 unloads the weapon and slides it across the ice so that it clatters against the rocks on the island's shore. They eventually cross the ice safely and retrieve the gun. Of course, they get nowhere near the ring-necks, who are long-gone, having flap-cackled their way across to the south side of the river without having to fool around with any silly self-control strategies such as making a Commitment Response.

Let's try an example of using the self-control strategy of making a Commitment Response to meet some goal that you might choose related to having prostate cancer. Since the most consistent dietary advice I have seen with regard to prostate cancer is the elimination of meat, I'll assume that many readers may choose that as a goal. Many will find this change in eating difficult. However, the use of a Commitment Response strategy can increase your chances of success.

Again, remember that a Commitment Response involves performing some behavior at one particular time that changes the likelihood that you will perform some other behavior at a later time. Imagine you are at the grocery store. What would a Commitment Response look like? Simple. When you are in the grocery store, DO NOT walk down, do not even glance, at the meat aisle. By doing so, you prevent the opportunity for the later choice between eating and not eating the meat once it is at home. It is much easier to avoid part of the grocery store than it is to fight off the temptation of food that is within the reach of your fork.

A person could even use such a strategy to ensure that he acted in accordance with his values regarding marital fidelity, as illustrated by the man in this poem.

VALUES AND BEHAVIORAL SELF-CONTROL

Commitment: Performing Behavior A at Time 1
to alter the probability of Behavior B at Time 2.

> 1170s B. C.—Ulysses lashed to the mast—
> 1960s—Payroll savings plan—
> 1974—Rose, a young woman,
> > among the few he's met whose
> > beauty rivals that of his wife,
> > offers him a ride home one Spring day.

Confession: like Jimmy Carter
he lusts in his heart
(and other bodily locations)
when her short skirt
sashays past his laboratory door.

Sliding in beside this siren,
he is still young and
possessed by enough arrogance
to imagine her invitation leading
them someday far beyond transportation--
thus, Behavior A (the Fib),
"I just remembered work I need to do in the
Psych Building; just drop me off here,"
which prevents . . . you know. . .
well, I guess it's a new term for it. . .
but . . . prevents . . . Behavior B.

November 2, 2009

The Premack Principle—Another easy-to-remember method of self-control was designed decades ago by a psychologist named David Premack. The Premack Principle formalized the fact that for any pair of actions, you could use the one that occurred more often as a reinforcer to strengthen the one that occurred less often. If you required the performance of the lower-probability action before allowing the performance of the higher-probability action, the former would occur more frequently in the future.

In an early application of this idea, Lloyd Homme and his colleagues (1963) were helping a nursery school teacher with her unruly class. Homme observed the children for a while and picked out a behavior that they seemed to spend a lot of time on when they were left to their own devices. The high probability behavior he chose to use as his reinforcer was running around the room and yelling. The behavior the teacher wished to strengthen was sitting quietly in their desks, an activity that was happening at a woefully low rate.

Homme set up a contingency whereby if the kids sat quietly for a certain amount of time, they were told they could get up and run and scream for a few minutes. The effect was dramatic. Time spent sitting quickly skyrocketed, so that even with the time spent running and screaming, more learning could take place.

Note that Homme didn't ask whether or not the kids liked to run around and scream. To employ the Premack Principle, all he had to do was find an activity that happened *more often* than the behavior of sitting quietly. Kid stuff? Could be, but I got through graduate school partly by taking advantage of the fact that eating chocolate chip cookies was a higher-probability behavior than studying.

This technique is available to you at any time, in any place. Just find a behavior that is more probable than the one you are having trouble doing, and set up a contract that makes this behavior available only after you have completed some amount of your target behavior, the less probable one.

Suppose you've thought it would be cool to build little chairs for each of your grandchildren. You've had the thought, but not acted on it, and the months and years have drifted by. Look around you. What do you spend a lot of time doing? What do you make certain to get done each day, no matter what? Ah-hah! That didn't take you long, did it? Well, in case it did, ask your spouse. I'll bet she can tell you.

Let's suppose that checking your email comes to mind. First thing in the morning, you log on. You check for messages numerous times during the day. You remember that when you were camping, you even went into town and hit a Starbucks to use their Wi-Fi on several occasions.

So now, combine making a Commitment Response and the Premack Principle to get those chairs finished (well, started first, since you have yet to measure a single board.) Take an 8 ½ X 11 inch piece of paper and write out a contract with yourself. "I will only check my email each day after I have spent at least thirty minutes building the grandchildren's chairs." Use a bright marker pen for your sign. Tape, tack, glue, pin, staple or nail this sign next to your computer, so that you can't avoid seeing it every time you sit there. Tell your wife about this contract. Tell your plan to all your kids and grandkids, your email friends, and the pals with whom you golf, bowl, fish, hunt, or drink beer. People's encouragement or harassment may help you reach your goal.

Recording Your Behavior—It's a great idea to use a calendar to keep track of what you are doing. Nothing fancy. For example, soon after I took up long-distance running in 1977, I began to record my running activity every day. I started with one of the dedicated running logs, but I soon opted for the Sierra Club or Wilderness Society calendars with the seven days of the week on one page and a stunning outdoors photograph on the facing page. I have gotten one of these calendars from the kids each Christmas for over 20 years. My recording has ranged from as simple as noting the number of miles I ran on a given day (with a zero put in for any day I didn't run) to an elaborate description of where, with whom and how fast I ran, what the weather was like, whether I bicycled or did some other sort of exercise, and how I felt after exercising.

For the last decade or so, I recorded each day the number of miles for the day, the cumulative number for the week, and the cumulative number for the year. While all this recording may seem obsessive, it helped keep me going. When I would see a series of zeros popping up, I would be motivated to get off my butt and out the door. I recently added up all the recorded mileage and found out that over the last 34 years, I have recorded a total of

51,598 miles run. Despite much searching, I have been unable to locate my diaries for 1989 and 2001, though I am certain I kept records those years and ran significant mileage, since I completed a 50-mile run both years. Also, after I had pneumonia in 1981, I stopped recording the last seven months of the year and recorded for only 57 weeks out of 104 in 1982 and 1983. Adding in even a conservative estimate of miles run during those periods puts me well over 55,000 miles, so I can say with confidence that I have circled the globe twice on foot. See what you get for being compulsive?

Before you go to bed, merely write down the number of minutes you spent building chairs each day. If you want to get fancy and still have a simple way to keep track of your chair-building time, do what I did in graduate school. I purchased a small, cheap alarm clock, cut the cord, and wired in a small toggle switch that I pilfered from the Psychology Lab. I mounted the clock right in front of me on my desk. Each morning, I set the clock at 12:00. Each time I sat down to study, I flipped the switch to ON, and the clock started running. I switched it to OFF whenever I daydreamed or got up for some reason (such as to go get some of those Premack-inspired cookies). I turned the switch back on when I resumed studying.

Of course, you don't really need the switch. You can plug and unplug the cord from the wall repeatedly, or just write down a running total of your time, but the switch was a reminder to me. At the end of each day, I noted the number of minutes and hours that the clock had run that day and recorded that figure on a graph, so that I could see my progress on an ongoing basis.

Silly? You may say I shouldn't have had to go through all that rigmarole. Maybe. On the other hand, I did complete my degree, and I still have a diploma that reads "Doctor of Philosophy in Psychology" sitting next to a red-orange alarm clock in a keepsake box in the basement. Note to self: You thought it was sitting down there. Then in June 2011, when you looked for it to help you focus your time to finish this book, it had disappeared among all the basement detritus.

The BUT/AND Technique—Steven Hayes is a Professor of Psychology at the University of Nevada at Reno. At a workshop years ago, I heard him describe another simple self-control technique called BUT/AND. This strategy uses the power of words to affect our actions.

I often ended a psychotherapy session with a homework assignment that my clients and I had created. This homework was an activity they would engage in before our next session. I soon learned that whenever they said "I'll try" with regard to completing this task, it meant that they were not really going to do it, but did not want to disappoint me by saying so. Instead, they would show up the next week and report failure to finish the assignment.

After a while I tried to "cut through the crap" by responding that, in my experience, "I'll try" meant just that—that they were going to "try," but not that they would do it. I would add, "It would be healthier for you simply to tell me that you really did not plan to follow this plan, and then we could talk about doing something else, or figure out how you might accomplish what we have agreed upon."

In a similar manner, clients would repeatedly meet my suggestions of more adaptive behavior by saying something such as, *Yes, I'd do that BUT . . . .* The BUT was always followed by some reason why they couldn't do it. It was as though the word BUT acted retroactively and made the prior action impossible.

Hayes encouraged people to learn to recognize when

they were behaving this way and make a change. Reverse the order of the two phrases, and switch the BUT to AND. For example, instead of saying to yourself, *I'd mow the lawn, BUT it's hot outside,* you would say, *It's hot outside AND I am going to mow the lawn.* Or change, *I'd visit my grandma at the nursing home, BUT it smells funny in there* to *It smells funny at the nursing home, AND I am going to visit my grandma there.*

If everyone waited until they felt like doing things before doing them, much less would get done in the world. If we were nice to our spouses only when they had done all that we desired, marriages would be even more troubled than they are. Much of what gets accomplished in the world happens in spite of the kinds of conditions that typically follow the word BUT. If I judged it appropriate with a particular client, I would suggest they get off their BUT.

BUT/AND is particularly useful in cases of very advanced cancer. At some point, trying to control anything significant with regard to the disease may be not only fruitless, but counterproductive. Some would say that Acceptance strategies work best here. It's valuable at such a time to remember that though there may be little outside of yourself, or within yourself in terms of the disease process, that you can control, you always have the opportunity to influence your behavior with something similar to BUT/AND.

So if you have metastasized cancer, you might find yourself thinking, *I'd go visit the grandkids, but I'm too depressed,* or *I'd help my wife plan the Christmas party, but I have to go through this therapy,* or *I'd work on that end table I am building, but I might be dead before I finish,* please give BUT/AND a chance. Reverse the order and change BUT to AND. For example, *I'm depressed, AND I am going to go visit the grandkids.*

Or suppose your PSA did not stay at zero after your

surgery, and you are procrastinating about your next PSA recheck. You might notice words running around in your head such as *I'd get that recheck, BUT I'm afraid that it has increased.* Okay, you do the BUT/AND on that one for practice. Then get in and have your blood draw.

Anyone who has learned to use self-talk techniques can put them into play to maintain the sorts of emotional reactions that add to the quality of their life, even while that life is fading away. In a similar manner, they can also do more of the things that would enhance their daily lives.

DOG ROPE EATRR—You've probably guessed that I like acronyms. They help me remember lists of things. From Mr. Trainor's introductory biology class in 1964, I still recall the qualities that something must have in order to qualify as an animal. Respiration, Excretion, Digestion, Growth, Irritability, Reproduction, and Locomotion—RED GIRL. No way would I remember that list of required characteristics 48 years later without that acronym as a mnemonic. Heck, I repeatedly check books out of the library or order movies from NetFlix® and read or watch large parts before I remember that I have already read the book or watched the film. Worse yet, a while back it took me three days to remember the name of the actress Michelle Pfeifer.

To sum up this section on self-management, I created the following acronym to give you ready access to the steps you can take to control your own behavior. Just remember DOG ROPE EATRR. Yeah, silly, I know, but look what RED GIRL did for me.

Behavior Self-management

1. **D**EFINE a target behavior you wish to change.
2. **O**BSERVE and record this behavior.
3. Set a **GO**AL with regard to this behavior.

4. Create a plan to **REWARD OR P**UNISH the target behavior.
5. Rearrange your **ENVIRONMENT** to make the target behavior easier or more likely.
6. **ELIMINATE** any **AUTOMATIC THOUGHTS** that interfere with the target behavior.
7. **R**EASSESS and **R**EPEAT these steps based on your progress.

Let me take you through an example of using DOG ROPE EATRR. Suppose you want to become more appreciative of the small, everyday things in life. Wow, that presents a problem. How do you DEFINE "appreciate" as a behavior? How about, I appreciate each time I stop and think about what I am experiencing and notice the feelings that are present? So if you are driving in your car, hurrying and worrying about getting to an appointment on time, you count an "appreciate" as noticing the clouds as they pass by, and focusing on your shoulders, causing you to relax a bit.

Maybe you can carry a 3X5 card in your pocket and make a hash mark each time you OBSERVE an "appreciate" and put the day's total on your calendar before bed. Or wear a wrist stroke counter used for golf.

You might decide that you want to reach a GOAL of 50 appreciates per day.

There's no sense trying to reach 50 the first day or week of your project. So begin with a smaller step of aiming for five the first day, and REWARD your efforts by putting a dollar in a jar each day you reach your goal, the money to be saved for something you have wanted for a long time. You can gradually increase the size of your goal to six or eight or more appreciates per day, until you reach 50. OR you could follow a similar strategy, but add a requirement that you PUNISH poor performance by subtracting a dollar each day you miss your goal.

Change the ENVIRONMENT around you to increase your chances of success. Suppose you make a half-dozen small signs that say AWARE and put them in places like your dash-board, your computer screen, and your bathroom mirror.

Notice if you are saying things to yourself that interfere with your progress. Sometimes, when people try to focus on their world, they get distracted by "hurry up" thoughts like *I don't have time. There are important things to do. It's a waste not to be productive all the time.* ELIMINATE these AUTOMATIC THOUGHTS by countering them with more reasonable ideas, so they don't get in the way.

At the end of the week, REASSESS what you have done so far and decide whether your progress is adequate, or whether you need to tweak your plan to increase its effectiveness as you REPEAT it for another week.

Now you do it.

If you get nothing else from this book, you should end up with a variety of ways to manage yourself to live more fully, whether you are gravely ill or perfectly healthy. The steps in the Seven Cs present an outline for change, with a bit more detail on managing moods. DOG ROPE EATRR guides you through a process of self-control slanted somewhat more toward changing your actions.

Each of these methods acknowledges the importance of changing both feelings and action. Pick and choose which one seems most applicable in a particular situation with a particular goal. Making a Commitment Response, employing the Premack Principle, and BUT/AND are three specific self-control methods that can help you do more of the things you want to do each day. Different ways to skin a cat.

People sometimes define freedom in terms of having

choices. If you do not have the skills to manage your behavior, you are less free; you can't take advantage of that freedom. The same is true if you are hamstrung by emotional overreactions. Self-control or self-management doesn't mean always being busy, always striving for goals, any more than having a car that can reach speeds of 125 mph means always driving fast.

Having self-management skills means you can choose. You can decide when to be busy and active, and when to be more slowed down and contemplative. Self-management can include deciding to do nothing, to be deliberately at rest, but it is a conscious choice rather than a drifting style of being at the whim of whatever life forces come along.

<u>Again, Don't Drift</u>—William Jefferson Clinton must have developed tremendous skills at managing his behavior to reach his many accomplishments. Of course, while I find much to admire about him, I wish he would have employed more effective self-management techniques at times during his career. For example, if Bubba would have had better impulse control, the 2000 election would probably not have been close enough to allow George W. Bush to be elevated to the presidency by the Supreme Court in place of Al Gore. Improved zipper management in the presence of Monica Lewinski would have prevented the ill-advised (to put it charitably) war in Iraq.

All that aside, I find Clinton's comments in a February 21, 2011, TV special with Chris Matthews titled: *President of the World: The Bill Clinton Phenomenon* to be relevant to the idea of drifting. Clinton alluded to his heightened sense of his own mortality after his heart attack. His views about the whirlwind activities of his retirement make a fitting conclusion to this section.

He reminds us that it is stupid to waste the life we do have by focusing on things we are no longer able to do. Instead, he said that after his heart attack, he has lived by the rule, "I'm just going to throw myself in heart and soul, have the best time I could."

Coping Versus Mastery Models of Behavior—I have found that people are quite curious about how psychologists live their lives, and how they deal with adversity. I think they often believe either that psychologists have everything figured out, as my clients often thought about me, or that we are all crazy, and that's why we went into the field of psychology in the first place.

When I was doing psychotherapy, I tried to present myself to my clients as a coping model, rather than as a mastery model. Research I read in graduate school (Meichenbaum 1972) compared a condition in which people watched a model who completed a task on the first attempt without errors, with one in which the models took several tries, working their way through a number of false starts and errors before finally succeeding. Anxiety reduction was the subject of the study. Subjects observing the coping models consistently showed greater reduction of anxiety than those watching the mastery models.

Thus, I chose to be more disclosing than are many other therapists about the ways in which I struggled with problems in my own life. I believe I did so in a limited, appropriate manner and tried to be certain that I was doing so to provide my clients with the benefit of a coping model, without trying to satisfy any needs of my own.

In years past, I think I may have come off as someone who handled things quite well without struggles, since when I later talked with friends from graduate school about issues that were worrying me, such as ventricular tachycardia and prostate cancer, those people indicated they felt closer to me because I was willing to share with them what was going on in my life. I hope that by talking openly about my own ways of dealing with having prostate cancer, I have presented you with a coping model that will help you do what you need to do to live well, with this or any other disease.

Summing Up

It might be useful to conclude by providing you with a short list of specific suggestions of things you can do to smooth your travel down the Prostate Cancer Road:

TEN THINGS TO DO TO DEAL WITH PROSTATE CANCER

1. Get a dog (or maybe a cat or an iguana or an emu).
2. Get moderate exercise nearly every day.
3. Create and maintain loving, supportive relationships with your friends and family.
4. Make your diet more like Asian or Italian diets, along with a minimum of meat and dairy and an emphasis on fruits, vegetables, nuts, and supplements that support your immune system. Drink some red wine in the evening.
5. Get appropriate medical checks in a timely fashion.
6. Accept, experience, and maybe even express whatever feelings result from having prostate cancer.
7. Implement CBT self-talk skills: (1) to weaken the exaggerated emotional overreactions that get in the way of living a full life, and (2) to strengthen the emotions and attitudes that promote such a life.
8. Don't drift through your days. Take control of those things you can control, and be the steward of your

own life, your own coach, choreographer, director, and producer. Set goals (Mini-Bucket List?) and use self-management techniques to promote actions and habits that define, for you, a life well-lived. Then work at letting go and accepting those things over which you have no control.

9. Try your hand at writing about what your disease means to you.

10. Look around you each day. Be glad that you have this day, and take time to appreciate the mystery and beauty of our world.

Did This Book Reach Its Goals?

Now that we are about finished, I ask you to reflect on your reading of this book. If I have accomplished five things, I will feel that I have done my job. Consider the following goals that I hoped to reach in the writing of *The Rancid Walnut*:

1. To help you learn something about the nature of prostate cancer, about its diagnosis and prognosis, about the complicated decision-making process regarding the various ways to treat the disease, and about the pros and cons of various treatment modalities;

2. To encourage you to feel whatever you feel with regard to your own disease or the disease of a loved one, and the freedom to express those feelings to people with whom you feel safe;

3. To put you on the pathway to improving skills to manage your emotions and your actions, so that you can avoid drifting and instead live the rest of your life as fully as possible;

4. To convince you to consider therapeutic writing. I invite you to sit down now and spend a few minutes writing about your experience with prostate cancer. Do

244 R. Steven Heaps Ph.D.

this whether it is you or a loved one who has the disease. You will probably get the most benefit from this exercise if you repeat it each day for several days and focus on your feelings, as well as on what you think about the cancer or how it changes your behavior. Don't worry about grammar or spelling or punctuation. This can be just for you. There is considerable evidence that this kind of writing is a beneficial activity, even if no one else ever reads what you have written. On the other hand, if you wish to help me resuscitate my *Prostatus Poetica* project, send me your writing, and I will see if I can combine it with the work of others into a book that could benefit many men and their loved ones as they confront this common threat. There is great value in knowing that we are not alone.

5. And finally—not only because I am still one of the class clowns, but also because we know that "laughter is the best medicine" is more than just an old cliché—I hope that I have at least gotten you to chuckle a time or two.

With all the advances in the treatment of prostate cancer, there is great reason for hope. Make sure you remind yourself of the good fortune you have to live today.

Above all, remember that one of the major themes of this book has involved the idea of control. I have urged you to take control of everything that you can with regard to your disease, and in that way to counter a sense of helplessness and to let go of the aspects over which you can have little or no influence.

I want to remind you here that even if you reach a point at which you can exert no control over your disease, you still have a great deal to say about which actions you choose and what sort of internal dialogue runs through your mind. By managing your thoughts and your behaviors, you can minimize the amount of debilitating emotional overreactions that can detract from the quality of your life experience.

I think that following a cognitive-behavioral plan similar to this is a good idea for anyone, regardless of the status of their health.

I hope you have gotten some knowledge as well as some enjoyment from sharing my journey. Good luck to you as you travel down your own path.

APPENDIX

HOW IN THE WORLD DO YOU WRITE A WHOLE BOOK?

In the final chapter, I spoke about people being curious about how psychologists lived their lives. People are also curious about the details of the ways in which others go about this business of writing. I've never gone to a reading by an author at which, during the question and answer period, someone didn't ask questions such as: Where do you get your ideas? When do you write? Do you write each day? Where do you write? Do you use a computer? Do you follow an outline? Do you write quickly, then go back and rewrite, or do you self-edit as you go?

I won't wait for your questions. To begin, you already know that this book arose out of the for-now-abandoned *Prostatus Poetica* project.

Next, you should realize that there is another sort of meaning of the question "How do you write a book?" which can be translated as: "How in the world do you ever discipline yourself to stick with such a big task as to write a whole book?"

Though I will talk about this latter meaning of the question below, the quick answer is the same as the answer to the "How do you eat an elephant?" question I discussed earlier. I remember when I was beginning to write my Ph.D. dissertation. One of my committee members, Richard

Powers, whom I discussed in the self-control section, lived across the street. One night over a beer, he said, "Don't even think about writing a dissertation. Just think about writing the first chapter; that's all you are doing—then go on to the next part." Again, I followed the strategy of one step at a time, and I ended up with a 160-page document with 121 references, which was acceptable to my committee, and that's the bottom line.

When it came to the actual writing of this book, I used three main tools: spiral bound notebooks that I buy by the dozens when they are on sale for a dime before the school year starts, a miniature digital recorder, and my laptop computer. Probably over one-third of the material was first scribbled out in the notebooks.

Quite frequently, I had great ideas about writing when I awakened in the night. After staying awake, trying various mnemonic schemes to carry my thoughts into the morning light, I finally gave up and kept a notebook with a pen attached to it on my nightstand. Writing in the dark made for some interesting deciphering, but I usually was able to transform the nocturnal rough draft into something on the laptop that I could use.

Joe Henderson is a very accomplished long-distance runner, and the author of numerous books and monthly columns for *Runner's World* magazine. In talking about his writing, he described a routine of running for an hour each morning, allowing thoughts to simmer in his consciousness, then sitting down to write.

My writing ideas, more often than not, were first captured while I was walking, running, or riding in the car. Sometimes I would leave myself a message on our home answering machine with my cell phone, so that I would not forget what I was thinking. More often, I immediately grabbed a notebook when I came in the door and made a few notes.

After a while, I found myself following a routine similar to Joe Henderson's, though not with the sort of regular discipline he maintained. In the past, I would be running and think of something, trying to remember it till I got home, only to forget that creative idea. Then my daughter gave me a digital recorder—in fact, this note about the digital recorder was recorded on the digital recorder while I was running.

Unfortunately, when I was finishing this note the first time, I hit the wrong button and erased the prior nine notes that I hadn't transcribed over the last few days. I hope they weren't too important. At least memory cells, the structures that encode memory in the human brain, are amenable to recovery of lost information, at least some of the time. Not so, the digital recorder.

Of course, I carried on some of my usual routines that drive my wife nuts. That is, I had many of the notebooks lying around with several pages of writing on each, and I would rummage among them, or worse, ask her where a certain one might be. Over time, my organization improved. To her surprise, I actually created separate computer files for different chapters and labeled at least some of my notebooks.

The poems in this book were written over a three-year period, quite a few in our travel trailer on the Oregon Coast. I kept no particular schedule and wrote somewhat episodically. Most of the first draft, by the way, was written with almost no editing. I was just putting words down, though divided roughly by chapters that seemed appropriate. Massive rewriting followed, of course.

Writer's Block

Many people complain of Writer's Block, the special case of procrastination in which a person is unable to get words down on paper. Procrastination, in general, is often costly, yet it is rampant. One might ask how such a maladaptive pattern could continue. Where's the payoff for this behavioral style? The prevalence of procrastination makes more sense when you focus on the relative power of the short-term and long-term consequences of behavior that I discussed under self-control.

Again, we, just like other animals, are very susceptible to the immediate, or shorter term, consequences of our actions. We usually procrastinate about doing things that take effort and activities that we do not expect to enjoy. We substitute activities that bring a quicker payoff. Thus, we need strategies to overcome our habit of putting things off until later, especially when we take on a big task such as writing a book.

I used several methods to counter procrastination. Early on, I began charting the number of words I had written, using a table that listed number of words written for each chapter and an overall total. I frequently checked my tally and set informal goals for the next week or month.

Soon, I just monitored the total number of words in the entire manuscript. Microsoft Word gives you a very easy way to keep an ongoing tally with the Word Count function. I don't know that the code-writing geeks at Microsoft thought of it when they set up this function, but they created an easy way for a writer to strengthen his or her own writing behavior by clicking on Word Count and seeing day-to-day, even moment-to-moment, progress. And as I say this, I am reminded that I don't even have to click on anything, because in the lower left corner of my screen, it says, "Page 83 of 90, Words: 41,948."

Now this might seem childish. A mature adult, especially one with a Ph.D. in psychology, for goodness sakes, shouldn't have to go through all these machinations in order to get himself to sit his butt down and do what he needs to do, right? Well, the reality is that psychologists, as well as everyone else, need to find ways to manage their behavior to reach their goals. If it takes simple recording of behavior and even more involved reinforcement and punishment contingencies to get the job done, so be it.

In using such techniques to motivate me to keep writing, I joined a select group of authors. Joe Pear was my friend and colleague at the University of Manitoba. He regularly taught a course using Skinner's *Verbal Behavior* (1957) as a text. I believe it was when preparing for this course that Pear came across a wonderful book by the novelist Irving Wallace, entitled *The Writing of One Novel* (1968.) In this work, Wallace takes the reader on a journey that follows the writing of his blockbuster bestseller, *The Prize*.

Wallace opens a revealing window into the work of writing a novel, from the origin of the idea, through extensive research, the agonizing outlining and preparation of character notes and plot details, through the nitty-gritty details of the long grind of putting thousands of words on paper, and the ongoing give and take with a literary agent, publisher, and editor.

Pear was intrigued by Wallace's use of recording his various work activity. Just as I did, Wallace kept a chart which tracked the number of pages he wrote each day. He included copies of the charts for the writing of *The Prize*, beginning with a five-page day on October 19, 1960, and finishing with the final page, number 1,115, at 6:29 p.m. on February 24, 1961. Wallace also sent Pear copies of his diaries for the writing of *The Plot* and *The Man*, the last of which included notations of days off from writing, such as on the days of John F. Kennedy's assassination and funeral. Pear went on to show similarities between this writing behavior and the behavior of pigeons, rats, and people in laboratory settings under particular schedules of reinforcement.

Wallace stated that he didn't know why he originally started tracking his writing behavior in this manner, but he did so from very early in his career. I find his speculations in this regard insightful. He suggests that because he was on his own as a freelance writer, he needed to create some artificial structure that would bring some discipline to his work. He believed that the chart on the wall worked for him by providing both guilt and encouragement.

He avoided revealing to others that he used such techniques, fearing that he would have been considered odd or unprofessional. Later, he discovered that numerous other authors of renown had also been word or page counters, including Anthony Trollope and Ernest Hemingway, who wrote down his daily word count on the side of a cardboard box directly under the nose of a mounted gazelle head. Heady company, indeed.

I recently found a copy of Wallace's *The Writing of One Novel* in a used bookshop. To my delight, I discovered that Wallace also regularly used other behavioral strategies to help him overcome procrastination. He referred to one such method as a game. Put simply, to get himself going in the absence of ready-made external forces, he announced to the important people in his life that he was starting to write his book. In this way, he says he ". . . put my pride on the line, a promissory note that must be paid in the future." (p. 26) Sounds like a Commitment Response to me.

I followed a pattern similar to that described by Wallace as I wrote *The Rancid Walnut*. First, I did not tell even Karen until I had been writing for several months. It was another year before I began telling a few select people. When I did tell others what I was doing, I was using a "Commitment Response" strategy: doing something at Time A (making a formal statement about my goal) that increased the probability that I would do something else at Time B (continue writing until I finished). This strategy helped me to persevere, even during those periods when I did not want to write, and those days when I would read what I had written and engage in detrimental self-talk, such as *This is crap. No one is going to want to read your narcissistic blathering.*

Here is a paragraph I wrote last summer.

Hey, here I am on June 22, 2011, and my word count just turned to 63,533. I wrote over 700 words this morning, only because I sat down and began even when I really wanted to go outside and run on the trail along the river in the sunshine. Now I'm going for that run (reinforcement, right?) I remember when I thought it would be a great feat if I could get to 30,000 words, so maybe some of these self-control techniques have worked. P. S. Now three months have passed and I've added another 10,000 words and am finished with my first complete draft.

It is now the 19th day of February, 2012. The Word Count at the bottom of my computer screen reads 75,529, and I am finished with this puppy. I even have a contract to publish it, and this final draft is being emailed to the publisher today. Good for me!

GLOSSARY

AAA—see abdominal aortic aneurism.

Abdominal aortic aneurism—a bulging out of the wall of the major artery from the heart to the lower part of the body usually associated with a weakening of the wall of the artery.

Ablation—the therapeutic destruction of body tissue, often with radio-waves.

Adenocarcinoma—a malignant tumor arising from secretory cells in the epithelium.

Alexithymia—a condition in which an individual is to varying degrees unable to identify his or her emotions.

Anastamosis—the connection where the ends of the urethra have been sewed back together after the prostate is removed during surgery.

Anatomical (nerve-sparing) surgery—method devised by Patrick Walsh for removal of prostate gland while leaving the cavernosa nerves intact, thus preserving erections.

Androgen suppression therapy—use of female hormones to inhibit male hormones that facilitate growth of prostate cancer cells.

Apoptosis—"cell suicide;" a process through which cells kill themselves.

Atalectasis—a condition in which the lungs are partially deflated and contain excess fluid.

Atrial fibrillation—an abnormally rapid heart rhythm originating in the lower chambers of the heart.

Benign prostatic hyperplasia—non-cancerous enlargement of the prostate gland which inhibits urination through constriction of the urethra.

Beta-blocker—class of medications most often used to control high blood pressure; also useful for arrhythmias.

Betapace—trade name for beta-blocker drug sotalol.

Biochemical failure—an increase in PSA level following prostatectomy or radiation treatment; suggests cancer cells may still be present.

Biopsy—removal of tissue for analysis, e.g., for the presence of cancer.

Brachytherapy—radiation therapy in which radioactive pellets or seeds are implanted in the prostate.

BPH—see benign prostatic hyperplasia.

BUT/AND method—a self-control method for overcoming procrastination.

Capsule—the outer wall of the prostate gland.

Catheter—a drainage tube; after a prostatectomy, a catheter allows urine to flow out of the bladder through the anastamosis without leaking into the body cavity.

Cavernosa nerves—the nerves, located along the edges of the prostate, which are "spared" in nerve-sparing surgery.

CBT—see Cognitive-behavior therapy.

Cognitive-behavior therapy—a school of psychotherapy which uses analysis and modification of thinking and direct behavior-change strategies to alter emotions and actions.

Commitment response—a self-control strategy in which a person performs one behavior at an earlier time to alter another behavior in the future.

Computerized tomography—computerized diagnostic imagining using X-rays to show cross-sectional views of the body.

Conditioned suppression—a disruption in ongoing behavior in the presence of something that has been associated with an unpleasant event.

Coping versus mastery model—two ways of presenting information to be imitated: one in which the model makes and then corrects errors, and another in which the model performs flawlessly.

Corpora cavernosa—spongy structures within the penis which become engorged with blood to produce an erection.

CT scan—see computerized tomography.

Cyberknife®—a robotic radio-surgery system which uses a computer-controlled arm to deliver radiation from a variety of directions to different parts of the prostate.

Digital rectal exam or rectal exam—a procedure in which a physician examines the prostate gland for palpable abnormalities by inserting a lubricated finger into the rectum.

DRE—see Digital rectal exam.

DOG ROPE EATRR--acronym for a set of steps for managing one's own behavior.

EBRT—see External-beam radiation therapy.

External-beam radiation therapy--cancer treatment which sends X-rays from outside the body to inside the body (e. g., to the prostate) to attack cancer cells.

Free radicals—atoms or molecules that contain an unpaired electron; promote oxidation and increase DNA damage and tumor growth.

Functional MRI—a magnetic resonance imagery study that depicts biological activity by means of measuring blood flow.

Gleason score—method of rating the amount of disorganization of the structure of cancer cells; higher scores suggest a more aggressive cancer.

GST-π enzyme (glutathione-S-transferase-π enzyme)—a "scavenger" enzyme that combats free radicals and protects cells from damage caused by oxidation; is increased by consuming cruciferous vegetables.

Gynecomastia—abnormal enlargement of the breast in a male.

Immune system—a complicated set of cells, tissues and organ through which the body recognizes and fights invaders.

Intensity-modulated radiation therapy—an external-beam radiation therapy that uses numerous individual beams to more closely match the radiation dosage to the shape of the prostate.

Kegel exercises—a regimen of repeated contraction of the pubococcygeus muscle to improve urinary control.

Learned helplessness—the phenomenon of an organism failing to escape or avoid a preventable aversive event due to a history of the same event being uncontrollable.

Locus of control—a concept which purports to represent the degree to which people believe they can (internal locus of control) or cannot (external locus of control) influence events in their lives.

Magnetic resonance imaging—an imagining technique using a magnetic resonance scanner rather than X-rays to create cross-sectional views of the body.

Margins—see surgical margins.

Metastasis—the spread of cancer beyond the organ in which it originated.

Mitral valve—the valve between the left atrium and the left ventricle of the heart.

MRI—see Magnetic resonance imaging.

PET scan—see Positron emission tomography.

Positron emission tomography—an imaging method which uses radioactive isotopes to view biological activity in cross-sections of the body.

Premack principle—a statement that for any two behaviors, the one that occurs more frequently can be used to reinforce the frequency of the less frequent one.

Prostascint® scan—a specialized radioactive examination that evaluates whether PSA-containing cancer cells have metastasized following treatment for prostate cancer.

Prostate gland—in males, the small gland surrounding the urethra and located below the bladder; this gland produces most of the seminal fluid.

Prostate specific antigen—see PSA.

PSA—prostate specific antigen; an enzyme produced by the prostate gland in response to a variety of factors, such as infection, as well as in response to a malignancy. Its level is commonly measured as an initial screen for prostate cancer.

> bound PSA—PSA that is chemically joined to other proteins: higher amounts suggest a higher probability of cancer.

free PSA—PSA not chemically joined to other proteins: free PSA arises almost entirely from tissue that causes the non-malignant disorder called benign prostatic hypertrophy; higher amounts suggest less likelihood of cancer.

Proton therapy—a computer-guided radiation treatment for prostate cancer that uses protons rather than photons (as with X-ray based approaches). Adherents claim comparable results and fewer side effects than X-ray based methods, though others question this claim.

Velocity of PSA—a measure of how fast a man's PSA is changing over time.

Psychoneuroimmunology—the study of the influence of psychological factors on the functioning of the immune system through the mediation of the neurological system.

Rational emotive therapy—a school of psychotherapy created by Albert Ellis, in which the emphasis is on changing irrational thinking to change emotion and behavior.

Rectal exam—see Digital rectal exam.

Regurgitation—leaking, as when a defective heart valve allows blood to flow backwards from a ventricle to an atrium.

RET—see Rational emotive therapy.

Salvage radiation—radiation therapy performed after there has been a rise in PSA following prostatectomy.

Seven Cs method—a method for changing emotion and behavior.

Sotalol—a beta-blocker drug which has specific anti-arrhythmic properties.

Staging—the process of using measures such as PSA, PSA velocity, imaging studies, and digital rectal exam to estimate the severity of prostate cancer.

Surgical margins—the outermost edges of tissues removed in surgery.

> negative margin—a surgical margin in which no cancer cells are found.

> positive margins—a surgical margin in which cancer cells are found.

Tenormin®—a beta-blocker drug.

Three-D CRT therapy—a type of radiation therapy using advanced imagining techniques to deliver numerous X-ray beams to provide more precise targeting of prostate tumors.

Ventricular tachycardia—an abnormal, rapid heart rate arising in the left ventricle of the heart.

Watchful waiting—a strategy of repeated testing, e.g., by PSA measurements, postponing surgical or radiation treatment of cancer until test results meet some criteria of severity.

REFERENCES

Beck, A. T., Rush, A. J., Shaw, B. E. & Emery, G. *Cognitive Therapy of Depression.* New York: The Guilford Press, 1979.

Beyers, D. Proton therapy for prostate cancer: show me the CER! (cancernetwork.com, June 15, 2008.)

Blum, R. H. & Scholz, M. *Invasion of the Prostate Snatchers.* New York: Other Press, 2010.

Boyles, Salynn. PSA Screening Guidelines Stir Debate. *WebMD Health News,* 27 April 2009.

Bill-Axelson, A., Holmberg, L., Ruutu, M. Haggman, M., Andersson, S. O., Bratell, S., Spangenberg, A., Busch, C., Nordling, S., Garmo, H., Palmgren, J., Adami, H. O., Norlen, B. J., Johansson, J. E. Scandinavian Prostate Cancer Group Study No. 4. Radical prostatectomy versus watchful waiting in early prostate cancer. *New England Journal of Medicine,* 2005, 12, 1977-84.

Burns, D. D. *Feeling Good: The New Mood Therapy.* New York: Wm. Morrow and Co., 1980.

Catania, A. C. Freedom and knowledge: an experimental analysis of preference in pigeons. *Journal of the Experimental Analysis of Behavior,* 1975, 24, 89-106.

Cohen, L. Parker, P. A., Vence, L., Svar, C., Kentor, D., Pettaway, C., Babaian, R., Pisters, L., Miles, B., Wei, Q., Wiltz, L., Patel, T., & Radvani, L. Presurgical stress management improves postoperative immune function in men with prostate cancer undergoing radical prostatectomy. *Psychosomatic Medicine*, 2011, 73, 218-225.

Cousins, N. *Anatomy of an Illness as Perceived by the Patient*. New York: W. W. Norton, 1979.

Doig, I. *Winter Brothers*. Boston: Houghton-Mifflin, 1982.

Dreher, M. Pomegranates and Prostate Health: A research report. prostate cancer research institute (www.prostate-cancer.org) Aug, 2008.

Ellsworth, P. Heaney, J. & Gill, G. *100 Questions & Answers About Prostate Cancer*. Boston: Jones and Bartlett Publishers, 2003.

Epplein, M., Zheng, Y, Zheng, W, Chen, Z., Gu, K., Penson, D., Lu, W., & Shu, X. O. Quality of life after breast cancer diagnosis and survival. *Journal of Clinical Oncology*. 2011, 29, 406-12.

Fantino, E. *Behaving Well*. Atlanta, GA: Performance Management Publications, 2007.

Farwell, W. R., D'Avolino, L. W., Scranton, R. E., Lawler, E. V. and Gaziano, J. M. Statins and prostate cancer diagnosis in a veterans population. *Journal of the National Cancer Institute*, 2011, 103, 885-892.

Frias, M., Pereira, & Ibanga, I. Imus said stress may have provoked cancer. abcnews.go.com (*Good Morning America*), March 17, 2009.

Frankl, V. E. *Man's Search for Meaning*. New York: Simon and Schuster, 1963.

Gilbert, D. *Stumbling on Happiness*. New York: Vintage Books, 2005.

Gladwell, M. *The Tipping Point*. Boston: Little, Brown and Company, 2000.

Gladwell, M. *Blink*. Boston: Little, Brown and Company, 2005.

Gottman, J. *Why Marriages Succeed and Fail*. New York: Simon and Schuster, 1994.

Gould, S. J. The median isn't the message. *Discover*, 1985, 6, 40-42.

Greenberger, D. & Padesky, C. A. *Mind Over Mood: A Cognitive Therapy Treatment Manual for Clients*. New York: The Guilford Press, 1995.

Grippando, James. *Intent to Kill*. New York: HarperCollins, 2009.

Homme, L. E., deBaca, P. C., Devine, J. V., Steinhorst, R. & Rickert, E. J. Use of the Premack Principle in controlling the behavior of nursery school children. *Journal of the Experimental Analysis of Behavior*, 1963, 6, 544.

Jacobs, A. J. *The Year of Living Biblically*. New York: Simon and Schuster, 2008.

Johnson and Johnson Incorporated. 2010 Annual Report.

Kabat-Zinn, J. *Mindfulness for Beginners*. Sounds True, Inc., 2006.

Kabat-Zinn, J. *Coming to Our Senses: Healing Ourselves*. New York: Hyperion, 2007.

Kipper, S. Update on ProstaScint®: CT and MRI fusion as diagnostic tools. *Prostate Cancer Research Institute Insights*, 6, #3.

Kenfield, S. A., Stampfer, M. J., Chan, J. M., & Giovannucci, E. Smoking and prostate cancer survival and recurrence. *Journal of the American Medical Association*, 2011, 305, 2548-2555.

Klein, E. A., Thompson, I. M., Taugen, C. M., Crowley, J. J., Lucia, M. S., Goodman, P. J., Minasian, L. M., Ford, L. G., Parnes, H. L., Gaziano, J. M., Karp, D. D., Lieber, M. M. Walther, P. J., Klotz, L., Parsons, J. K., Chin, J. L., Darke, A. K., Lippman, S. M., Goodman, G. E., Meysken , F. L., Baker, L. H. Vitamin E and the risk of prostate cancer: The selenium and vitamin E cancer prevention trial (SELECT.) *Journal of the American Medical Association*, 2011, 306, 1549-1556.

Kubler-Ross, E. *On Death and Dying*. New York: Scribner, 1969.

Kushner, H. *When Bad Things Happen to Good People.* New York: Avalon Books, 1981.

Lehrer, J. *How We Decide.* New York: Houghton-Mifflin, 2008.

Meichenbaum, D. H. Examination of model characteristics in reducing avoidance behavior. *Journal of Behavior Therapy and Experimental Psychiatry*, 1972, 3, 225-227.

Nyguen, P.L., Trofimov, A., & Zietman, A. L. Proton-Beam vs. Intensity-Modulated Radiation Therapy. *Oncology*, 22, 2008.

Ornish, D., Weidner G., Fair, W. R., Marlin, R., Pettengill, E. B., Raisin, C. J., Dunn-Emke, S., Crutchfield, L., Jacobs, F. N., Barnard, R. J., Aronson, W. J., McCormac, P., McKnight, D. J., Fein, J. D., Dnistrian, A. M., Weinstein, J., Ngo, T. H., Mendell, N. R., & Carroll, P. R. Intensive lifestyle changes may affect the progression of prostate cancer. *Journal of Urology.* 2005, 17, 1065-1069.

Paddock, C. Prostate Cancer Guidelines for PSA Screening, *Medical News Today*, (www.medical newstoday.com) 27 April 2009.

Penedo, F. J, Antoni, M. H, & Schneiderman, R. *Cognitive-Behavioral Stress Management for Prostate Cancer.* New York: Oxford University Press, 2008.

Pennebaker, J. W. *Opening Up: The Healing Power of Expressing Emotions*. New York: Guilford Press, 1997.

Psychological Stress and Cancer: Questions and Answers, National Cancer Institute FactSheet, 4/29/2008, http://www.cancer.gov/cancertopics/factsheet/Risk /stress.

Rachlin, H. & Green, L. Commitment, choice and self-control. *Journal of the Experimental Analysis of Behavior*, 1972, 17, 15-22.

Roberts, K. J., Lepore, S. J., & Helgeson, V. Social-cognitive correlates of adjustment to prostate cancer. *Psycho-Oncology*, 2006, 15, 183-192.

Rodin, J. & Langer, J. E. Long-term effects of a control-relevant intervention with the institutionalized aged. *Journal of Personality and Social Psychology*, 1997, 35, 897-902.

Roth, P. *Exit Ghost*. New York: Houghton Mifflin Co., 2007.

Rotter, J. B. *Social Learning and Clinical Psychology*. New York: Prentice-Hall, 1954.

Rush, J. M., & Hussain, M. H. Evolving therapeutic paradigms for advanced prostate cancer. May 16, 2011 posting of *Oncology*, volume 25, #6 article on cancernetwork.com— pages not shown.)

Schachter, S. & Singer, J. E. Cognitive, social, and physiological determinants of emotional state. *Psychological Review*, 1962, <u>69</u>, 379-399.

Schover, L. R., Canada, A. L., Yuan, Y., Sui, D., Neese, L., Jenkins, R. & Rhodes, M. M. A randomized trial of internet-based versus traditional sexual counseling for couple after localized prostate cancer treatment. online issue of *Cancer*, September <u>26</u>, 2011.

Schwartz, B. *The Paradox of Choice*. New York: HarperCollins Publishers, 2005.

Segerstrom, S. C. & Miller, G. E. Psychological stress and the human immune system: A Meta-Analytic Study of 30 Years of Inquiry. *Psychological Bulletin*, 2004, <u>130</u>, 601-630.

Seligman, M. E. P. *Learned Helplessness*. San Francisco: W. H. Freeman and Co., 1975.

Seligman, M. E. P. *Learned Optimism*. New York: Alfred A. Knopf, 1991.

Seligman, M. E. P. *Authentic Happiness*. New York: Simon and Schuster, Inc., 2002.

Skinner, B. F. *Science and Human Behavior*. New York: McMillan, 1953.

Skinner, B. F. *Verbal Behavior*. New York: Appleton, Century Croft, 1957.

Sklar, L. S. & Anisman, H. Stress and cancer, *Psychological Bulletin*, 1981, <u>89</u>, 369-406.

Stein, R. Diet, Exercise and Reduced Stress Slow Prostate Cancer, Study. *The Washington Post*, August 11, 2005.

Steinmetz, J., Blankenship, J., Brown, L. Hall, D. & Miller, G. *Managing Stress Before It Manages You*. Palo Alto, California: Bull Publishing, 1980.

Stone, A. A. Stress and social support linked to prostate cancer. Posted on www.cfa.org, September 21, 199.

Tolmunen, T., Lehto, S. M., Heliste, M., Kurl, S., & Kauhanen, J. Alexithymia is associated with increased cardiovascular mortality in middle-aged Finnish men. *Psychosomatic Medicine*, 2010, <u>72</u>, 187-191.

Torrey, E. F. *Surviving Prostate Cancer*. New Haven: Yale University Press, 2006.

Unknown author. Stress may help cancer cells resist treatment, *ScienceDaily*, April 11, 2007.

Voltaire. *Candide*. New York: Bantam Books, 1959 (original edition, 1759).

Voss, S. C., & Homzie, M. J. Choice as a value. *Psychological. Reports*, <u>26</u>, 912-914.

Wallace, I. *The Writing of One Novel*. New York: Pocket Books, 1971.

Wallston, K. A., Wallston, B. S. & DeVelis, R. Development of the multidimensional locus of control (MHLC) scales. *Health Education Monographs*, 1978, <u>6</u>, 160-170.

Walsh, P. C. & Worthington, J. F. *Dr. Patrick Walsh's Guide to Surviving Prostate Cancer*, New York: 2001.

Walsh, P. C. & Worthington, J. F. *Dr. Patrick Walsh's Guide to Surviving Prostate Cancer, Second Edition*. New York: Wellness Central, 2007.

Wilson, K. M., Kasperzyk, J. L., Rider, J. R., Kenfield, S., van Dam, R. M., Stampfer, M. J., Giovannucci, A. & Mucci, L. A. Coffee consumption and prostate cancer risk and progression in the health professionals follow-up study. *Journal of the National Cancer Institute*, 2011, <u>103</u>, 1481.

Withers, B. *BraveHearts*. Chicago: Triumph Books, 2002.

Zilbergeld, B. *The New Male Sexuality*. New York: Bantam Books, 1992.

CPSIA information can be obtained at www.ICGtesting.com
Printed in the USA
BVOW012355090412

287271BV00004B/1/P